Diabetes and You

Diabetes and You

A Comprehensive, Holistic Approach

Naheed Ali

ROWMAN & LITTLEFIELD PUBLISHERS, INC.
Lanham • Boulder • New York • Toronto • Plymouth, UK

Published by Rowman & Littlefield Publishers, Inc.
A wholly owned subsidary of The Rowman & Littlefield Publishing Group, Inc.
4501 Forbes Boulevard, Suite 200, Lanham, Maryland 20706
http://www.rowmanlittlefield.com

Estover Road, Plymouth PL6 7PY, United Kingdom

British Library Cataloguing in Publication Information Available

Library of Congress Cataloging-in-Publication Data

Ali, Naheed, 1981–
  Diabetes and you : a comprehensive, holistic approach / Naheed Ali.
    p. cm.
  Includes bibliographical references and index.
  ISBN 978-1-4422-0728-8 (cloth : alk. paper) — ISBN 978-1-4422-0730-1 (electronic)
  1. Diabetes. 2. Diabetes—Alternative treatment. 3. Holistic medicine. I. Title.
  RC660.A45 2010
  616.4'62—dc22   2010029235

Printed in the United States of America

Diabetes and You is dedicated to my students, to diabetics, and to all of you who provided encouragement and support throughout this project.

Contents

viii   *Contents*

Disclaimer

Diabetes and You represents reference material only. It is not intended as a medical manual, and the data presented here is meant to assist you in making informed choices regarding your wellness. This book is not a replacement for treatment(s) that may have been suggested by your personal physician. If you believe you are experiencing a medical issue, it is recommended that you seek professional medical help. Mention of particular products, companies, or authorities in this book does not entail endorsement by the publisher or author.

From the Author

$\mathcal{T}$his book shows how diabetes patients can have a chance to enjoy a satisfying life if proper care is taken. Through self-control and the right management techniques, patients can persevere in the struggle against this dangerous illness, which in modern times can lead to several other chronic diseases now affecting people all over the world. Statistics show that over the last twenty years the number of people worldwide afflicted by diabetes has risen from 30 million to 246 million! I can affirm that this "silent killer" gradually erodes the wellness of its victims. Having no fear of disease can at times be the best way to fight off diabetes, and through specific considerations relating to health, a diabetic can benefit from a healthy lifestyle through practice and commitment.

To begin with, reflect on your own habits (diet, exercise, and other activities) and the habits of those close to you. If you do the research, you will realize that people with chronic renal failure (a long-term kidney disease) often trace the root cause of their disease to diabetes. Unsteady nutritional habits, lifestyle, and other aspects of your health history (for example, frequent drinking, smoking, and eating fatty foods) all contribute to dangerous conditions.

Patients with chronic renal failure because of diabetic complications undergo dialysis to cleanse the blood of the wastes accumulated in the liver. All of this may have originally started from diabetes, and because of a simple intolerance to glucose, other vital organs of the body may be impacted. Instead of enjoying a healthy life, diabetics have to endure many restrictions in what they eat, drink, and do in everyday life.

It is commonly stated, "Once a diabetic, always a diabetic." But is this really true? As we continuously combat this disease, and while trying to avoid it myself, I cannot help but think how lifestyle changes would help more people. Instead of just sitting and watching diabetes ruin their lives, with greater consciousness and awareness of what can be done, we can offset diabetes by working consistently against it.

Diabetics can be empowered to use their own capabilities to work for wellness. I have encountered many diabetic patients suffering from a wide range of symptoms, and I know that this disease can be ultimately overcome. Patients who have taken control of many of their hardships stand as living proof that this disease is a tower that can eventually be climbed.

Diabetes and You will help you get a handle on the basics of what you need to know about diabetes and will help you understand the whys and wherefores of the illness, diagnosis, and treatment. If you are aware of the various implications this disease has for the whole body (particularly the mental and cardiac effects), you will understand why you need to intensify your knowledge about diabetes. Like other dreaded ailments, diabetes has a huge impact on both the mind and body of the individual in question. When you are dealing with someone who has diabetes, make a few observations. You might notice the mood swings, frustrations, and grieving that he or she undergoes. A diabetic usually feels sad, questioning why he or she has diabetes. In turn, family members who observe the emotional turmoil in their loved one often become upset as they misunderstand the diabetic's situation.

What can be done to support someone who has these problems? Based on behavioral and mental approaches, the best means is to provide adequate support. In order to promote a therapeutic environment for the patient, you have to employ effective communication.

When journeying through *Diabetes and You*, we will discover the wide spectrum of approaches available to you in addition to effective communication. You won't really need a psychotherapist to provide treatment or necessary support. In the end, there is always something you can do personally to alleviate symptoms of the disease. Use this book to help you look diabetes right in the eye and face it in the most commanding way.

When it comes to diagnosis and insulin therapy, you will encounter familiar terms, such as the types of diabetes, designated as Type 1 and Type 2 diabetes. Type 2 diabetes is easier to detect since the afflicted people are usually obese. We can also easily distinguish the difference between Types 1 and 2 based on factors such as age. For the most part, Type 1 diabetes affects young people, which is why it is called juvenile diabetes. In recent years, however, Type 1 diabetes has also been found in adults in the form of latent autoimmune diabetes. Some of the medications and treatment protocols mentioned in this book as part of the overall management of a diabetic can be very expensive. For example, insulin is an absolute need for many with diabetes, and it requires considerable financial resources. With all of the symptoms and financial commitments involved, the diabetic must inevitably realize that the overall fight against the disease takes time and adjustment. Diabetes isn't something that vanishes overnight. The diagnosis, symptoms, and overall management of the disease are not always a straightforward and easy process to go through.

The patient says, "Diabetes?! I'm doomed!" The acceptance process takes time. It may even require substantial changes in lifestyle. As a result, the diabetic may experience changes in mood and mental fragility, thus keeping him or her from experiencing life to the fullest. Patients may also suffer from mood swings, which can lead to misunderstandings with family members and caregivers, thus adversely affecting important interpersonal relationships.

Negative emotions are just a sprinkle in the sea of problems a diabetic may encounter, and they can also indicate underlying physical pain. Various types of pain afflict the diabetic, which in turn may lead to emotional and physical frailty. Common complaints include headaches and nerve pain accompanied by other symptoms, such as vision abnormalities, kidney issues, and nerve damage. If you observe the pathophysiology (the effects of the illness on the body) of diabetes, you might not notice these complications in a diabetic right away. But, one by one, they will gradually manifest themselves. Yet, with proper diagnostic procedures, such as urine tests and constant monitoring of blood glucose levels, many of the complications associated with diabetes can be avoided.

People in today's self-help obsessed society are constantly talking about diet. By reading this book, you will gain insights into the foods you should avoid and those you need to have in significant amounts. If you are a diabetic who loves to cook and bake pastries, consider whether what you are preparing is really good for your health. If you have a tremendous love for sodas, consider the amount of sugar you are putting into your body. In chapter 9, you will be introduced to a handful of factual guides that demonstrate which foods you should or should not eat.

In what ways can diabetes pose major problems for diabetics who are trying to properly manage themselves and their families? Is there a reason why more and more people are suffering from this dreaded killer in modern times? Over and over, I ask, what can be done? Do we ingenuously watch and pretend nothing is happening? We have to wake up! Many are already affected. Why wait for your time to come?

Kudos to all physicians and other health care providers who are promoting preventive measures for diabetes throughout the community, as it is necessary to recognize the health care professionals who devote their time and passion to caring for the sick. Besides the physicians and nurses who do their part in treating the disease, what can diabetics themselves do to take action against diabetes? There are many ways to respond to such a question, and I hope the following chapters will provide the answers that diabetic patients need.

Part One

DIABETES AT A GLANCE

• 1 •

Diabetes Explained

$\mathcal{P}$eople tend to think of diabetes as the presence of high blood sugar levels in the body, which requires people to follow a strict diet and take insulin shots. But just what exactly is diabetes? Why do people say it is one of the enemies of good health? Take a deeper look into what experts call the "illness of the rich."

Diabetes used to be known as *insulin dependent diabetes mellitus* (IDDM) and *noninsulin dependent diabetes mellitus* (NIDDM). These terms are not used as commonly today because of the possibility of confusion for those who aren't familiar with the medical jargon. Instead, we now use the terms *Type 1* and *Type 2 diabetes* (Arabic numerals are preferred over Roman numerals to avoid any possible confusion).

Being metabolic (that is, involved in breaking down consumables and converting them into energy), diabetes is an outcome of the processes that take place when the body digests food. When we eat, food is changed into glucose, the form that sugar takes when it is "active." This serves as the main source of fuel for our bodies. The glucose then goes into the bloodstream and passes through the rest of the body for energy and growth. For glucose to reach the cells, the body uses insulin, a hormone secreted by the pancreas. The pancreas is the large gland found at the back of the stomach.

Statistics show that 5 to 10 percent of diabetics have Type 1 diabetes, in which beta cells do not produce enough insulin, thus requiring insulin injections for the patient. Type 1 diabetes is like the hijacking of immune processes whereby the body's own cells attack themselves. These destructive autoimmune processes eventually lead to illnesses like diabetes mellitus and other autoimmune disorders (e.g., Crohn's disease, Goodpasture's syndrome). Type 1 diabetics are usually diagnosed before the age of thirty. Type 2 diabetes

3

occurs gradually, meaning that it has a slow onset, and approximately 90 to 95 percent of diabetics have this kind. This form of diabetes happens due to insulin resistance or sensitivity. It can cause impaired functioning of the beta cells which leads to reduced insulin production.

At first, Type 2 diabetics are prescribed common remedies, such as diet and exercise. When blood glucose levels continue to escalate, physicians may prescribe oral hypoglycemic agents. *Hypoglycemia* means low sugar in the blood. In some individuals suffering from sudden stress, the medicines don't work, which leads to a serious need for insulin injections. Type 2 diabetes typically afflicts people who are obese and over the age of thirty.

Complications occur not only for those who take insulin. Whatever the type of diabetes, the patient's condition can unfortunately spiral out of control once the individual's body is affected by different factors that lead to complications. With proper management of the symptoms and avoidance of factors that trigger specific symptoms, diabetics can steer clear of life-threatening complications.

Type 2 diabetics may have the impression that they do not actually have diabetes simply because they don't take insulin injections. They believe they have "borderline" diabetes, but this idea is potentially harmful for them. Diabetics must take their conditions seriously, follow the doctor's advice, and learn alternative means for preventing symptoms and avoiding complications.

If you are a health care provider, you must be committed to educating your patients about the real picture. In doing so, you must urge them to work for their own wellness and help them to understand that what they have is not "borderline" diabetes but the real deal itself. Type 2 diabetes is also referred to as insulin resistance, impaired glucose tolerance (IGT), or impaired fasting glucose (IFG), a state wherein blood glucose levels act like an elevator and go up and down between average levels and those of a true diabetic.

HISTORY OF DIABETES

For centuries, people have studied diabetes and the underlying factors that lead to the illness. Today, much advanced research goes into the prevention and treatment of the disease. Insulin has been used to manage diabetes only since 1922.

Diabetes can be indicated by the occurrence of glucosuria, or the condition of having glucose in the urine. Ancient Hindu writings told of black ants and flies that were found lingering around the urine of those with diabetes.

Sushruta, an Indian doctor who lived around 400 BC, wrote about the urine of diabetics and described it as a sweet substance. Later on, physicians believed that sweet urine was a sign that a person had diabetes.

In 250 BC, the term *diabetes* was coined. Diabetes in Greek means "to siphon," as the disease was believed to drain an individual of fluid. The Greek physician Aretaeus explained that diabetics were being drained of their body fluid because they urinated more often than usual, and he vividly described the disease as the "liquefaction of flesh and bones into urine." In 1674, King Charles II's personal physician, Thomas Willis, coined the term *diabetes mellitus*, with *mellitus* meaning "honey." Willis also believed a diabetic's urine was sweet or "imbued with honey and sugar."

In the 1800s, many different treatments were suggested for diabetics, including bloodletting and opium. Different diets were also suggested. In the early decades of the century, starving oneself was said to be an effective therapy. Sufferers were said to enjoy a longer life span through these practices. The treatment of diabetes took a major step forward in the late 1800s, when two German physicians, Joseph von Mering and Oskar Minkowski, removed the pancreas of several dogs and discovered that the dogs gradually developed diabetes. Through this discovery, the physicians tried to link the pancreas to diabetes and aimed to isolate a pancreatic extract that they hoped could treat the disease.

In Canada, Dr. Frederick Banting was eager to isolate the extract in spite of skeptics who didn't believe it could be done. In May 1921, Dr. Banting, together with his assistant Charles Best, a medical student, began experiments at the Toronto laboratory of Professor John Macleod. Banting tied off the pancreatic ducts of dogs to observe the behavior of insulin. The pancreatic cells, which release digestive enzymes, degenerated, while the cells that released insulin did not. After a few weeks, the pancreas disintegrated into sediment to the point that insulin could be isolated and retrieved. In July 1921, a dog with its pancreas removed was injected with extract obtained from another dog with tied ducts. As a consequence, the canine's blood glucose level dropped. Following this experiment, another dog with its pancreas removed was injected with the extract for eight days. The scientists observed the same results and called the substance "isletin."

The isletin studies caused the dogs to have lower blood glucose levels, thus improving their overall condition and causing their urine glucose levels to go down. It was observed that as long as the dogs received isletin, they survived. Later on, different animals were experimented on, with many experts now experimenting on cows rather than dogs. The animals could survive without a pancreas for a period of seventy days. This breakthrough led to improved diabetic research.

Following these experiments, Dr. James Collip, a biochemist at the University of Western Ontario, tried to develop a new extract with longer-lasting effects. On January 11, 1922, a fourteen-year-old boy named Leonard Thompson was the first to receive insulin injections. However, these injections produced only a slight decline in glucose levels and caused protruding abscesses at the site of the injection. Because of these unsatisfactory results, Dr. Collip worked on refining the insulin extract. After several weeks, the same boy was given the purified extract, and soon his health improved. His blood sugar levels were now up to par. He gained weight and managed to live another thirteen years, dying at twenty-seven from pneumonia.

During the spring of 1922, Charles Best continued to produce insulin to help in the recovery of patients at the Toronto clinic. For almost sixty years, insulin was manufactured to produce long-lasting, positive effects and became a flexible therapy for diabetic patients with evolving needs. In 1978, a change came about with the creation of recombinant human DNA insulin; instead of using animals, the substance could now be replicated from insulin produced by human beings. This was a major medical milestone.

In 1923, Macleod and Banting were awarded the Nobel Prize in Medicine for the discovery of insulin. They maintained that insulin was not actually a cure for diabetes but rather a treatment. Due in part to their experiments, it is now known that insulin helps metabolize carbohydrates and other nutrients that provide the body with energy for everyday activities.

TRACKING THE RATES OF DIABETES

According to the International Federation of Diabetes, the number of diabetics has grown from 30 million twenty years ago to more than 246 million today. Based on their statistics, seven of the ten nations with the largest number of diabetics are developing nations, with two of the nations being China and India. Most countries with a striking density of diabetics are located in the Middle East and the Caribbean.

The Centers for Disease Control and Prevention (CDC) suggests that 21 million Americans, or 7 percent of the total U.S. population, have diabetes. The big news is that, astonishingly enough, one-third of them don't have a clue that they have the disease. About 41 million Americans are currently prediabetic or are at high risk for contracting the disease. When prediabetes is left unmanaged, it can mature into Type 2 diabetes, and possibly cardiac disease.

In 2006, as determined by the International Diabetes Federation, diabetes was announced as the sixth leading cause of death in America. They also reported that 21 percent of those aged sixty and above are close to developing diabetes. Among twenty- to thirty-nine-year-olds, 2 percent are likely to develop the disease, followed closely by 10 percent of forty- to fifty-nine-year-olds.

According to the American Diabetes Association, at least 23 million people in the United States today suffer from diabetes. Of this number, about 17 million have already been diagnosed, while approximately 5.7 million have not.

The United States spends around $132 billion for this disease, with $92 billion being direct medical costs and the rest being in productivity losses and other costs.

As overwhelming as U.S. diabetes statistics are, compared to Third World countries, the situation is still manageable. In African and Asian countries, where insulin is very difficult to come by, diabetics may live only for two years or less following diagnosis.

Factors that lead to diabetes include unhealthy lifestyles, poor diets, and heredity. People nowadays exercise less and perform fewer physical activities, which prompts obesity. This causes stress on the system and the organs and makes the body unable to produce insulin.

If you have diabetes, you will slowly realize that, apart from the health predicaments you face, you could also be confronted with considerable economic hardships. There are treatment expenses and other health care costs, such as hospitalization, which is common in diabetics aged sixty-five and above. Diabetics are also more prone to life-threatening complications. The overall estimated costs incurred by diabetics in the United States, including direct and indirect expenses, may reach up to $100 billion each year. The aim of treatment regimens is obviously not a financial one, but is rather to bring down sugar levels to a suitable range, with the goal being to prevent acute and chronic complications.

There are more diabetics in developed nations because most of the people in these nations eat food that is rich in carbohydrates, which includes glucose. Foods like these lead to insulin resistance and are a key factor leading to Type 2 diabetes.

THE INNER WORKINGS OF DIABETES

Diabetes doesn't just suddenly appear out of the blue; nor does it make a person feel ill overnight. Prior to the disease taking shape, the body will have been exposed to various factors that encourage insulin intolerance. It is very important to learn about the pathophysiology and mechanism of diabetes. These are the processes that occur inside your organs and body systems once you are afflicted with the disease.

Let's begin with insulin. Since impaired insulin production is the main cause of diabetes, it is important to know its basic function. Insulin comes from beta cells, which in turn come from the islets of Langerhans located in the pancreas. As an anabolic substance, insulin builds molecules through the energy it receives from various sources. It also serves as a storage facility for glucose in the form of glucogen in the liver and muscles. When a person eats, insulin levels jump up, forcing glucose to move from the blood into the muscle, then to the liver, and in due course into fat cells.

Insulin serves the body by transporting and metabolizing glucose for energy, thus stimulating the storage of glucose. It signals the liver to halt the release of glucose, thus enhancing fat deposits in adipose tissue and accelerating the movement of amino acids from dietary protein to the inside of cells.

Insulin prevents stored glucose, protein, and fat from being degraded. Between meals and overnight, the pancreas releases very minute amounts of insulin, called the basal insulin rate. After blood glucose levels have been lowered, another hormone called glucagon is released from the pancreas by the alpha cells located in the islets of Langerhans. Glucagon causes the liver to secrete stored glucose and works with insulin to achieve typical sugar levels.

The liver manufactures glucose chiefly by breaking down glycogen through a process called glycogenesis. Once eight to twelve hours have passed without eating, the liver builds up glucose by breaking down amino acids and other noncarbohydrate substances via a process called gluconeogenesis.

Once insulin secretion is impaired in the pancreas, gastrointestinal (pertaining to stomach and intestines) absorption of glucose boosts basal hepatic glucose production in the liver and decreases insulin-stimulated glucose uptake in the muscles. Hyperglycemia then appears, indicating diabetes.

For Type 1 diabetes, the process is pretty much the same, but there is a genetic predisposition in Type 1 patients that causes beta cell destruction. This is explored further in upcoming chapters. For now we should focus on the basics.

ANATOMY AND PHYSIOLOGY INVOLVED IN DIABETES

In order to understand the processes that take place when a person has diabetes, it is important to learn about the organs and systems affected.

Foremost is the pancreas, which is found in the upper abdomen. It performs both endocrine (secretion of somatostatin, glucagons, and insulin into the bloodstream) and exocrine (release of enzymes in the intestinal tract via the pancreatic duct) functions.

During the exocrine function, the pancreas secretes enzymes from the pancreatic duct, which then pass through the connecting bile duct and enter the small intestine through an entrance area called the ampulla of Vater. Near the ampulla is the sphincter of Oddi, which controls the rate at which secretions from the pancreas and gallbladder enter the small intestine through the duodenum. The duodenum is the initial part of the small intestine.

The enzymes secreted from the pancreas by the exocrine function are digestive enzymes, rich in protein and filled with electrolytes. They are considered alkaline because they have high contents of sodium bicarbonate. This makes them capable of neutralizing acidic gastric juice as it enters the duodenum.

There are several different kinds of exocrine pancreas secretions. One of these is amylase, which aids in the digestion of carbohydrates. Trypsin is responsible for protein digestion. Lipase helps to digest fats. Other enzymes that help break down different food types are also active at this time.

Hormones from the gastrointestinal tract influence the secretion of exocrine pancreatic juices. The hormone secretin plays a major role in increasing secretions of bicarbonate from the pancreas. When speaking of digestive enzymes, the CCK-PZ hormone is the working hand.

Insulin, glucagon, and somatostatin are hormones that are active in regulating the body's stored enzymes and other substances that control the body's natural functions. The islets of Langerhans, the part of the pancreas involved in endocrine functions, is equally important. The pancreatic cells consist of alpha cells that give off glucagon, beta cells that give off insulin, and delta cells that produce the hormone somatostatin.

INSULIN VS. GLUCAGON

A primary role of insulin is to decrease blood glucose by allowing glucose to travel to the liver, muscle cells, and other tissues. The glucose is stored as glycogen and is otherwise used for energy. Insulin also allows for fat storage in adipose or fat tissue just as much as it synthesizes proteins in other body tissues. When insulin is low or absent, glucose is unable to move through the cells, and thus it exits the body in urine. Frequent urination is a symptom of diabetes mellitus. In the presence of diabetes, the body compromises and uses stored fats and proteins for energy purposes. This produces a loss of body mass. Glucose levels in the blood usually determine the rate at which insulin is secreted by the pancreas.

As opposed to insulin, glucagon's purpose is to reinforce total sugar levels by converting glycogen into glucose in the liver. The pancreas releases glucagon because there is a low blood glucose level. The somatostatin hormone produced by the cells in the pancreas interferes with the pituitary gland's secretion of growth hormone, which influences blood sugar.

INSULIN FROM A GENOMIC PERSPECTIVE

Scientists have spent many years researching insulin. Frederick Sanger of England led the way for research on insulin's genetic makeup and in 1958 determined the sequence of amino acids that constitute insulin. This was the first time that a certain protein had been discovered and its internal structure identified.

Insulin has two chains, chain A (with twenty-one amino acids) and chain B (with thirty amino acids), joined by two disulfide bridges. Generally speaking, the genetic makeup of insulin causes the chain length to be the same, and so the insulin from a pig can help a human with diabetes. Today, however, large-scale production of proinsulin developed through bacteria, or recombinant insulin, has replaced porcine insulin.

Insulin manufacture begins when a unique gene found at chromosome 11 is genetically translated, or activated. Preproinsulin is the main product of the translation. It has a signal peptide with twenty-four amino acids, enabling the protein to reach the cell membrane or boundary.

When the preproinsulin goes to a part of the cell called the endoplasmic reticulum, an enzyme called protease signals the production of proinsulin. In the endoplasmic reticulum, enzymes cause proinsulin to branch out and become mature and active insulin. Meanwhile, inside the Golgi body of a human cell, insulin is packed into secretory granules that form the cytoplasm of beta cells. This is why insulin is said to originate from the beta cells of the pancreas. The liver takes glycogen, the stored form of glucose, and converts it back to an active form when required.

DIABETES AND "STARVATION IN THE MIDST OF PLENTY"

Diabetes has been referred to as "starvation in the midst of plenty," since there are low levels of intracellular glucose while the extracellular levels are on the high side. During starvation, Type 1 diabetics rely on energy from sources beyond glucose, such as ketone bodies and fatty acids. Ketone bodies may be uncontrollable, and they cause major acidity of the blood. As a result, diabetic ketoacidosis (DKA) and hyperglycemia (increased blood sugar) follow.

In DKA, hypertriglyceridemia also occurs, and soon the liver mixes triglycerol and protein, forming very low-density lipoprotein (VLDL), which is then released into the circulatory system. In a diabetic, the low level of insulin linked to an elevated amount of glucagon paves the way to inhibiting the degradation of lipoproteins or lipoprotein lipase. If you have DKA, there's a good chance of high amounts of VLDL and chylomicrons coming from lipids in the diet.

INTRODUCTION TO THE DIABETIC DIET

Since the dawn of the twenty-first century, diets resembling the South Beach Diet and After Six have been created for the diabetic. These all boil down to restricting carbs in our meals.

In England during the 1860s, William Banting first stressed the effectiveness of low carbohydrate diets. Surpassing sixty years of age, Banting discovered that if he restricted carbohydrates, he would lose weight. In a single year, he lost forty-six pounds from his original weight of two hundred and two pounds. Banting thus stated, "Any starchy or saccharine matter tends to the disease of corpulence in advanced life." He reported that he was never hungry, and through effort he seemed to be more functional than ever. Eventually, a research study was undertaken involving thirty-six volunteers on low carbohydrate and low fat diets. It was initially found that a low carbohydrate diet led to speedier weight loss than a low fat one. At the end of the trial, however, the weight loss was the same in both diets.

A CLOSER LOOK AT NUTRIENTS

Since diabetes may stem from diet, we can grasp an idea of how the diabetic process begins if we learn about our food intake and the internal mechanisms that work as we eat. At the time when food is taken in, it is composed of fats, carbohydrates, and proteins. Later, these elements are broken down into particles (also known as constituent nutrients) that can be absorbed through digestion.

Carbohydrates are broken down into disaccharides, such as sucrose and maltose, and monosaccharides like fructose, glucose, and galactose.

Glucose, the main carbohydrate, is a major source of fuel for the body. It lets proteins become amino acids and peptides and makes fats shrink down to monoglycerides. Molecules are always easier for the body to metabolize when they are smaller in size.

Carbohydrates can be simple or complex depending essentially on size. Simple carbohydrates are tiny molecules that are easily absorbed by the body. An example is glucose, the key player in diabetes. Simple carbohydrates also supply energy faster than other sources because they are gentler and easier to break down. Carbohydrates quickly raise the level of blood glucose in the body because carbohydrates *are* sugars. Examples of foods that contain a large amount of simple carbohydrates are dairy products, honey, maple syrup, and fruits. Unquestionably, these simple carbohydrates provide the sweetness we taste in candies, cakes, and other sweet items.

Complex carbohydrates are made up of simple carbohydrates that are tied together and need to be broken down before the body can absorb them. Because they are difficult to absorb, they give energy much more slowly. However, complex carbohydrates still provide energy faster than proteins and fats. They also have less chance of being converted to fat, and they increase your sugars sharply and allow for carbohydrates to remain undigested for longer periods. Complex carbohydrates are present in fibers and starches, for instance wheat products like breads and pastas. They are also present in grains, corn, and rye, and in beans and root crops like potatoes and yams. Corn is indigestible because it contains so much of the complex carbohydrate called cellulose.

DIGGING DEEPER INTO THE FOODS WE EAT

Diabetics usually require significant modification of carbohydrates in their diet because *carbohydrate* is just another word for sugar. In diabetes, glucose is always the major carbohydrate (sugar) that is questioned among the vast number of other carbohydrates found in nature. Carbohydrates make up a major portion of the food a person eats, so it is important to know that there are two kinds of these giant molecules: refined and unrefined.

Refined carbohydrates are foods that have had the nutrients, fibers, bran, vitamins, minerals, and other components removed. This makes refined goods easier to absorb but less nutritious, since *refined* means "highly processed." Even when refined carbohydrates are fortified with vitamins and minerals later on, they still remain different in structure and function from unrefined ones. Refined carbohydrates have the same amount of calories as their unrefined counterparts, but they can grimly increase the risk of obesity and diabetes.

If carbohydrates are ingested in excess of the body's requirements, the body fails to convert energy in the proper way. Some carbohydrates will be converted to glycogen, while the rest will be turned into fats, resulting in weight gain.

Experts recommend that your total calories should account for 50 to 55 percent carbohydrates. The glycemic index (GI) of a carbohydrate tells how fast consumption really relates to high sugar levels. The index ranges from 1, which is the slowest rate, up to 100, the fastest, referring to pure glucose.

The human body doesn't depend exclusively on the GI to determine the rate of carbohydrate metabolism. To obtain more accurate results, take into consideration the type and amount of food you eat. Most complex carbohydrates have a reduced GI, and foods rich in fructose (fruit sugar) have a greater effect on blood sugar.

CARBOHYDRATE METABOLISM EXPLAINED

Glucose is derived all the way through the metabolism of ingested carbohydrates and proteins via gluconeogenesis (glucose production). It can also be temporarily contained as glycogen in the liver, muscles, and other tissues. The endocrine system regulates blood glucose levels by controlling the rates of synthesis, storage, and movement of glucose in the vascular system. The ideal level of glucose is around 100 mg/dL, or 5.5 mmol/L.

Insulin helps to bring down glucose levels. The hormone glucagon counteracts it, but so do epinephrine, growth hormone, adrenocorticosteroids, and thyroid hormone.

Concerning endocrine and exocrine processes, it can be noticed that the two mechanisms are highly related in terms of the functioning of the pancreas. The capacity of the exocrine pancreas is generally geared toward facilitating digestion by secreting enzymes into the proximal duodenum, the first part of the small intestine. Secretin and cholecystokinin-pancreozymin (CCK-PZ) are the hormones responsible for the digestion of substances from the gastrointestinal tract. They also aid digestion by mildly regulating enzyme secretions of the pancreas and other organs. Pancreatic dysfunction results in reduced enzyme secretions and impaired digestion of fats and protein. The healthy range of enzyme secretion from the pancreas gland is 1,500 to 2,500 milliliters per day.

GLUCOSE METABOLISM IN DIABETICS

Glucose tags along with insulin, so if you understand how this pairing works, you basically get the overview of how diabetes genuinely affects the patient. Let's take a closer look into glucose to understand how the body consumes and metabolizes the nutrients in food.

Though mostly the work of insulin, various hormones control glucose, and when you have a lot of glucose inside of you, insulin is readily secreted and supports a wide spectrum of other processes. Glucose is removed from the blood and transported to muscle and fat cells, where it is broken down as these cells release energy via adenosine triphosphate (ATP) in both glycolysis (the conversion of glucose to pyruvate) and citric acid cycle processes. Later, glucose is stored as glycogen in the liver and the muscles to function as an energy reserve in the short term. For long-term energy reserves, glucose is stored in adipose tissue as fat. Cells also utilize glucose and use its energy to make proteins whenever needed.

Sources differ when citing typical glucose levels. Some sources suggest 100 mg/dL, while others acknowledge 110 mg/dL. The average level of blood glucose is difficult to determine because the levels of blood sugar are never really constant. The ranges fluctuate depending on an individual's needs and the level of stress involved. Therefore, it is safe to say that more than one factor contributes to the rise and fall of glucose levels in diabetics. There are three main factors: diet (the more sugary foods you eat, the higher the level will be), the breakdown of glycogen, and the hepatic (liver) synthesis of glucose.

Glucose is a polar molecule, suggesting that it has both positive and negative charges attached to it. That is why there have to be specific glucose transporters (GLUTS) for glucose to be absorbed along with water into the gut wall. GLUTS come in various shapes and forms, and five types exist. The two most common forms are GLUT2 and GLUT5.

Where glucose metabolism is concerned, the liver is perhaps the most important organ to consider. It is one of the main structures of your body that produces sugar. The breakdown of glycogen produces glucose, which occurs when carbohydrates, fats, and proteins are thoroughly metabolized. The liver maintains levels of glucose by absorbing it from the blood. It accepts blood filled with glucose via the portal vein, connected directly to the digestive tract. When a person does not have diabetes, the liver gets rid of large amounts of glucose as the blood circulates, thus preventing a rise in glucose levels.

Prediabetes vs. Diabetes

Besides knowing about diabetes itself, it is also vital to know more about its precursor, known as prediabetes.

A person with prediabetes doesn't suffer from full-blown diabetes, but failure to manage the symptoms properly can drive him or her closer to Type 2 diabetes. Heart disease, already a major concern even for those without diabetes, is one major condition for persons with prediabetes to worry about.

A prediabetic patient will have insulin resistance very similar to that of a diabetic. In prediabetes, a patient cannot use insulin efficiently because of limited resources, so he or she has to compensate by trying to create as much new insulin as possible in order to reach appropriate sugar levels. Once a person has insulin resistance, abnormalities in fat and blood pressure occur. The arteries also get clogged up with plaque material made of cholesterol.

Managing Prediabetes

In managing prediabetes, efforts should be made to prevent full-blown diabetes and the cardiac diseases that might develop soon thereafter. Prediabetes combined with high blood pressure and elevated cholesterol levels is sometimes referred to as metabolic syndrome, or syndrome X. The body also has a very strong resistance to insulin when suffering from metabolic syndrome. It then tries to produce more insulin to make up for all that resistance, which is why people with syndrome X have a high risk for incurring full-blown diabetes.

Cause and Prevention of Prediabetes

Prediabetes is not a death sentence. With proper management, diabetes can be controlled, and those suffering from it may be able to live healthier and longer lives. Like diabetes, prediabetes can be prevented if its causes are understood. However, elevated glucose levels make a person more prone to developing diabetes and its complications.

The ordinary fasting sugar level (blood sugar amounts after dieting for a period of eight to twelve hours) is 100 milligrams per deciliter (100 mg/dL). Any amount beyond 100 is considered abnormal. To be considered prediabetic, the level must be between 100 and 125 mg/dL.

Avoiding high blood sugar levels is vital to your survival as a prediabetic. After years of continuously high levels of blood sugar, complications befall, including the following:

- Diabetic retinopathy (an eye disease)
- Nerve damage leading to amputation
- Impotence
- Diseases in the intestines
- Stomach problems
- Heart disease

- Bladder incontinence
- Kidney dysfunction

Prediabetes Risk Factors

Elevated glucose levels are also associated with high levels of fat (cholesterol and triglyceride) in our cells. This puts a prediabetic at greater risk for heart attacks, strokes, and other grave conditions. Risk factors for prediabetes are similar to the ones for diabetes itself, with obesity being the most prevalent.

There are statistical risk groups associated with diabetes, such as African Americans, Latinos, American Indians, and Pacific Islanders. People aged forty-five and above are at high risk, along with those with a family history of Type 2 diabetes. High blood pressure also immensely affects people with this illness.

Heart disease patients and people with elevated cholesterol levels are at risk for contracting prediabetes. Those with very low levels (40 mg/dL for men, 50 mg/dL for women) of "good" cholesterol (high density lipoprotein, or HDL) are also in danger.

Find a medical professional and seek out his or her advice if you suspect that you may have prediabetes. Ask yourself the following:

- Did you incur gestational diabetes or deliver a baby who weighed more than nine pounds?
- Have you been diagnosed with polycystic ovarian syndrome (PCOS), which causes insulin resistance?
- Do you dislike exercising on a regular basis?
- Has your doctor told you that you have impaired glucose tolerance or prediabetes?

A "yes" answer to any of these questions should signal a change to a healthier lifestyle.

INSULIN RESISTANCE IN MODERN MAN

A patient may experience insulin resistance even before he or she gets diagnosed with prediabetes or high sugar levels. As discussed by Dr. Anne Peters in her book *Conquering Diabetes*, insulin resistance is commonly labeled *metabolic syndrome*. With many diabetics having a parent with metabolic syndrome, the question, "Will I be at risk for metabolic syndrome?" is often asked.

If blood sugar is at unhealthy levels, the distribution of fat around the middle area of the body, the abdomen, makes an individual prone to developing diabetes. Moreover, elevated triglyceride levels and a decrease in HDL (good) cholesterol augments one's vulnerability to disease.

HOW TO TRACE THE PROGRESS OF DIABETES

To diagnose diabetes and prediabetes, a fasting plasma glucose (FPG) test or an oral glucose tolerance test (OGTT) is given to patients. As part of this screening, the diabetic drinks a bottle of bad-tasting liquid sugar. In the FPG test, a lab value of 100 to 125 mg/dL signifies prediabetes, while 126 mg/dL and above is deemed a positive diagnosis.

The blood glucose level is measured after fasting and again two hours after a glucose-filled beverage is consumed. If the level reaches 140 to 199 mg/dL, you are prediabetic, but if you have 200 mg/dL or more, then you are positive for either prediabetes or diabetes.

DIABETES AND STARVATION

The medical effects of starvation can be explained in terms of glycogen pathways and other body systems that work to enhance glucose production and other related processes. Starvation causes the liver to continually deplete all of the body's stored glycogen, thus encouraging the conversion of glucose from fats (glycerol) and from the amino acids in proteins.

Various organs utilize the energy that is produced when fatty acids are metabolized and broken down into acetyl-CoA (acetyl-coenzyme A). Within the citric acid cycle, ATP (adenosine triphosphate), which is a high-energy molecule, is generated as a major byproduct. When starvation persists, acetyl-CoA levels exceed the diabetic's oxidative capacity.

The liver reacts immediately by processing the fatty acids into ketone bodies so that the body will still have a source of energy. Because one of the organs, the brain, cannot metabolize fatty acids, it has to rely on ketones for energy. During the long and fretful days of starvation, the brain makes use of glucose to obtain the fuel needed to function well. After about two weeks of laboring without any nutrients, the brain starts using these ketones. Having too many ketones circulating around is grounds for DKA, as previously noted.

FURTHER INTRODUCTION

As a patient, you should never be afraid of diabetes. Everything you need to halt or prevent diabetes is readily available and at your disposal. It is also true that preventing is far better than curing. A healthy lifestyle is thereby the easiest way to avoid not only diabetes but other similar diseases as well.

Most diabetics can achieve a comfortable lifestyle these days, irrespective of their income levels. When everything you need is within arm's reach, there is no need to walk a mile to get what you want. With the rapid spread of advanced technology, people are increasingly able to perform the most arduous tasks from the comfort of their own living room. This makes it more difficult to stretch and exercise the muscles as a matter of routine.

It would seem that modernity itself has robbed people of healthy living, but this should not be the case if you determine your life based on your current and future health. You will always have the power to live according to your own choice. Choose to live a healthy life as a diabetic, away from the many temptations found in modern living.

· 2 ·

Types of Diabetes

$\mathcal{O}$nce you learn that you have elevated blood sugar levels, you are on your way to a restricted but healthier diet and lifestyle. You can also phase out diabetes and lessen its impact, given the necessary information about its types.

A deep discussion of the types of diabetes can equip you with essential knowledge about the prevention and treatment of the disease. When you get diagnosed with diabetes, your doctor should tell you immediately about the severity of your condition. The doctor might diagnose you with Type 1 diabetes, prescribe daily medication, and explain a bit about the benefits of using drugs to fight the disease.

Does this type of information really give you peace of mind, considering that you have this dreaded disease? You have the choice to be proactive and get all of the information you can get your hands on, but you must try your best to avoid becoming just another statistic in the hospital or diabetes clinic. This proactive mentality, which we will investigate further in upcoming chapters, is necessary for coping with diabetes.

TYPE 2 DIABETES IN A NUTSHELL

Type 2 diabetes is the most common form of diabetes. The most frequent causes of this type of diabetes are genetics, which can cause an innate deficiency in insulin production and the resulting failure to transfer sugar into cells, and lifestyle, including obesity, lack of exercise, and the like. Insulin dictates the breakdown of fats in cells and regulates the amount of fat and sugar flowing into the bloodstream. If there is excessive insulin, the blood

19

glucose level goes down. The opposite happens whenever the insulin level dives below average.

If your blood sugar level deviates from the standard quantities (usually 100 mg/dL), you may think nothing is wrong because of the absence of other symptoms. This is why diabetes is known as the "silent killer." In most instances, it is when you experience symptoms and complications that you acknowledge the severity of your situation. If you are insulin resistant, your blood sugar levels will eventually become difficult to handle.

In Type 2 diabetes, the insulin-providing beta cells of the pancreas "burn out" because of the unexpected demand that they produce more insulin. There are individuals with high rates of insulin failure, but their beta cells work adequately and thus they never suffer from diabetes.

The main characteristics of Type 2 diabetes are insulin resistance and impaired insulin secretion. Efforts to discover the causes of insulin resistance have not been fruitful to date, but to control the symptoms, insulin is necessary to regulate blood sugar levels and avoid the buildup of glucose. Once the beta cells are no longer able to produce enough insulin to keep up with the body's needs, Type 2 diabetes develops.

There may be impaired insulin secretion, but there may still be an adequate reserve of insulin to avoid the breakdown of fat and the production of ketone bodies. As a result, diabetic ketoacidosis (DKA) generally fails to take place in this type of diabetes. When DKA is reckoned uncontrollable, other related complications can quickly arise.

Type 2 diabetes primarily affects obese individuals over thirty, as noted earlier. Nowadays, younger individuals are developing this type of diabetes. With the insidious onset of glucose intolerance signals, many of these patients are surprised to learn that they even have diabetes.

Signs and symptoms of Type 2 diabetes are usually mild. These manifestations include the following:

- Irritability
- Fatigue
- Excessive thirst (polydipsia)
- Frequent urination (polyuria)
- Poor healing
- Skin wounds
- Blurred vision
- Vaginal infections (when there's too much glucose)

Knowing additional conditions related to Type 2 diabetes can provide an effective approach to handling your primary disease. One such approach is to keep a hawk's eye on your blood glucose level. With the various treatment alternatives available, positive outcomes are very likely if you constantly monitor your sugars. If you curtail your high blood sugar level too vigorously, though, you might end up with hypoglycemia, or insufficient blood glucose levels.

For you to know how hypoglycemia works, you have to understand the signs and symptoms that may affect your body. The most common warning signs are as follows:

- Excessive sweating
- Shakiness
- Dizziness
- Paleness
- Hunger
- Abrupt changes in mood
- Jerky movements
- Seizures
- Tingling sensations in the mouth

Have your blood sugar tested on a regular basis. To pull out of hypoglycemia, you need to take at least one of the following: three glucose tablets, a half cup of fruit juice, or five to six pieces of hard candy. Always consult your doctor first, as this is a very important element in conquering your disease. You must always carry some sugar snack with you in case you need it.

After fifteen to twenty minutes of primary intervention, check your glucose again. If it still hasn't gone up, repeat the treatment method until your blood sugar normalizes. If you pass out, you will need emergency treatment with glucagon or some other treatment that undeniably increases the amount of sugar in your blood.

Remember that insulin, food, and fluids should not be given to someone who has passed out. A fainted patient's hands should always be moved away from his or her mouth.

People who do not know that they have hypoglycemia suffer from hypoglycemia unawareness. Most individuals with this kind of hypoglycemia are chronic diabetics with nerve damage or neuropathy, patients whose glucose levels are strictly controlled, and people who are on medication for heart complications. To prevent or reduce hypoglycemia, it is very important for you to be informed about this condition so that your blood sugar can be monitored, your diabetes can be managed, and you can live a healthier life.

Hyperglycemia, a complication of diabetes and a primary symptom, can get seriously out of hand if not managed well. Hyperglycemia occurs when there is inadequate insulin in the body, specifically in Type 2 diabetics. There are instances when there is just enough insulin, but the insulin is unregulated and may even lead to hypoglycemia. Eating too much, failing to exercise, being under stress, and having other illnesses that affect your optimum functioning may bring on the above complications over time.

Hyperglycemia is easily diagnosed by various factors, including polyuria and polydipsia. Blood and urine tests provide information on the amount of glucose present in both. Frequent monitoring of your blood glucose levels is usually a good way to go. Ask your physician about the frequency of monitoring to have an idea of how to handle your condition and prevent the occurrence of additional difficulties. As soon as you learn that you have hyperglycemia, it must be treated.

If you are not successful at managing this condition, it could lead to ketoacidosis or diabetic coma, which are brought about by having too many ketones. When fats are broken down due to insufficient insulin, ketones are produced. Too many ketones in the circulatory system interfere with the body's ability to function properly. These ketones are partially eliminated in the urine, but it's really impossible to get rid of them all. They can accumulate very fast, eventually leading to ketoacidosis. Ketoacidosis is an emergency condition, characterized by shortness of breath, nausea, vomiting, fruity smelling breath, and dry mouth.

Exercise reverses a high sugar level in the body, but with glucose measurements greater than 240 mg/dL, the urine should be tested for ketones because continuing to exercise will lead to hyperglycemia. This is why it is important to consult your doctor about the right diet and exercise.

Besides the conditions already mentioned, diabetics can unfortunately also develop hyperosmolar hyperglycemic nonketotic syndrome (HHNS). HHNS affects older diabetic patients and can surface in both Type 1 and Type 2 diabetes, but it is more frequently associated with Type 2. It develops as a result of overwhelming symptoms and could have a serious impact on the diabetic's later health. In this dangerous scenario, your glucose level rises, leading your body to remove excessive amounts of sugar through urination.

Initially, persons with HHNS will experience polyuria (frequent urination) which eventually subsides and causes the urine to turn dark in color. HHNS also leads to constant thirst, which can lead to ion dehydration. Poor management of this condition can result in coma, seizures, and death. It is necessary to learn about the warning signs of HHNS to prevent any of this from happening. A blood glucose measure of more than 600 mg/dL, a dry mouth, warm dry skin, extreme thirst, high fever, weakness on one side of the body, hallucinations, loss of vision, and sleepiness are all signs of HHNS. The best way to avoid HHNS holistically is to monitor blood sugar levels, which many diabetics do every day between meals.

Approximately 75 percent of patients are diagnosed with Type 2 diabetes during a routine laboratory examination or a visit to the eye doctor. If left undiagnosed and untreated, long-term complications will arise in the form of peripheral neuropathy, eye disease, and peripheral vascular disease.

Obesity is one of the main factors leading to Type 2 diabetes, and weight loss is the immediate recommendation for defeating it. To enhance the effectiveness of insulin, you have to incorporate exercise into your treatment program. If exercise is unsuccessful, oral antidiabetic agents can be given, depending on the condition of the patient.

Likewise, insulin may be added to the regimen or administered alone. Some patients require insulin continuously, while others only require it when they are acutely stressed (usually during surgery or illness).

Since medications can delay the onset of the disease and its complications, they are widely used in today's society to suppress Type 2 diabetes. When you learn that you have Type 2 diabetes, don't panic when trying to figure out what medications will be best for you—that's the physician's job. Remember that once you are armed with information about your condition, as long as you uphold a healthy diet, exercise regularly, and obey your medical regimen, you will be much happier as a diabetic.

TYPE 2 DIABETES: RELATED CONDITIONS

The symptoms, prognosis, and manifestations of Type 2 diabetes may resemble other illnesses. Let's describe what other diseases have in common with diabetes.

Hemochromatosis

This is a single-gene illness characterized by the collection of iron in the tissues of the body. If left untreated, it can cause diabetes. Hemochromatosis is also termed *bronze diabetes* because it elicits a distinct discoloration of the skin.

One in two hundred Americans have the gene responsible for this disease. Half of these are expected to have medical difficulties. These rates are very similar to those of Type 1 diabetes, which, like Type 2, often goes unreported. Physicians advise that their diabetic patients have frequent blood tests to alleviate this problem.

In hemochromatosis, the single-gene mutation causes iron overload from the food in the intestines. Then the body cannot excrete iron as it normally does. Once this extra iron reaches the pancreas, liver, or the heart, serious damage may result without much notice.

People with hemochromatosis usually experience joint pain, fatigue, abdominal pain, loss of libido, and cardiac disease, as well as other diabetes symptoms. These symptoms usually happen in men aged thirty to fifty and in women aged fifty and above. The victims are also mostly overweight, but you obviously don't have to be overweight to suffer from these symptoms.

To detect high instances of iron, a serum ferrite test or transferring saturation test may be conducted. The genes may also be siphoned and analyzed to look for the specific one responsible for hemochromatosis. Owing mostly to symptom neglect and the scarcity of these tests, iron overload is often left untreated. This is when hardships arise. Some physicians mistakenly focus on other manifestations such as liver disease, heart conditions, arthritis, and diabetes and miss the iron overload, thereby keeping the cause of the hemochromatosis hidden.

A defective HFE gene is the principal cause of hemochromatosis. This gene is responsible for regulating the amount of iron we absorb from our food. Diabetics with homozygous genes, in which both parents have the defective gene, may inherit this disease. You are considered genetically "homozygous" if you have the same allele (two genes located in same position on a chromosome) on both chromosomes.

Blood tests are required for managing hemochromatosis. Diabetics generally have their blood tested once or twice a week for several months. When the iron level goes down, testing can be done every two to three months. Unlike diabetes, proper holistic evaluation and management can ease hemochromatosis symptoms. Suggested iron levels can be achieved after a series of blood tests have been completed. Once iron levels are managed, severe complications of the heart, liver, and other organs can be prevented.

Frozen Shoulder

Experts are currently debating whether diabetics are at serious risk for frozen shoulder. In this illness, also called adhesive capsulitis, the shoulders stiffen to the extent that swinging them while moving becomes quite a task. Once a shoulder is in pain, there is a tendency to stop using it, period. Diabetics with chronic shoulder pain prefer not to move their joints at all, sadly allowing the shoulder to lose mass and function.

Frozen shoulder accounts for underlying conditions like bursitis, which is the inflammation of the fluid-filled sac found in many joints. It can also result from tendonitis, which is inflammation of the tendons, and it can sometimes be a complication from stroke. Though these factors can contribute significantly to frozen shoulder, the real cause of frozen shoulder remains a holistic challenge. The medical community is still in the process of studying the connection between diabetes and this disease. There is a theory, however, that collagen, a major part of the ligament that holds the bones together to form a joint, has something to do with it. We think that glucose molecules bind to the collagen and lead to its accumulation in the cartilage and tendons of the shoulder.

According to numerous studies, 20 percent of diabetics and 5 percent of nondiabetics have frozen shoulder. Men and women between the ages of forty and sixty are more prone to frozen shoulder. This condition usually involves the weaker shoulder, and holistic treatment depends on the severity of the case. In the early stages of this condition, doctors usually advise conservative treatments like physical therapy. In the later stages, surgery is recommended.

Agent Orange

Agent Orange is not a disease but the code name for a herbicide used during the Vietnam War to defoliate trees and bushes. It was used to kill plants and leaves that served as hiding places for the enemy. Based on research with people who were exposed to this chemical, there could be a link between Agent Orange and Type 2 diabetes.

Vietnam War veterans and agricultural workers who used the herbicide were tested for dioxin, the suspected contaminant in Agent Orange. Results suggested that exposure to this chemical causes insulin resistance, the main symptom that occurs in Type 2 diabetes.

What exactly did scientists use Agent Orange for? Through animal testing, researchers discovered that dioxin and dioxin-like compounds (DLCs) cause illnesses like cancer.

In 1978, Vietnam War veterans underwent testing and were asked questions related to their exposure to Agent Orange. Their medical histories were taken, and laboratory tests and physical examinations were conducted. However, no concurrent and specific tests dealt with Agent Orange. Based on a 1994 report, only the levels of dioxin were identified in relation to Type 2 diabetes. This really doesn't allow any conclusions to be drawn, considering the unstable nature of dioxin metabolism and the large amounts of measurement error that were later found.

The various complications involved in each type of diabetes should be considered carefully, since the processes involved may deviate from one type to another.

For starters, you may want to investigate cardiac disease and stroke. According to the American Diabetes Association, two out of three diabetic patients die from heart complications. As a diabetic, it is vital for you to take preventive measures to avoid any general heart issues. Monitoring your blood pressure and cholesterol levels is paramount!

Above and beyond cardiac complications, the kidneys may also be affected as diabetes advances to a multiorgan dilemma. How does diabetes cause renal (kidney) problems? We need to focus on the loss of the kidneys' function, normally regarded as the filtration of toxins and waste products. As long as proteins, carbohydrates, and fats are digested, waste products will be created. The kidneys, which contain capillaries with microscopic holes, filter out a vast amount of waste products. These waste products are then expelled through urination. When protein and red blood cells are too large to pass through, they collect in our fluids.

In diabetics, for whom the blood glucose level tends to run high, the kidneys' workload increases because it is filtering an unusual amount of fluid. The malfunction tires the filters and causes leakage. As a result, proteins normally used by the body are wasted and passed out via urine. Having a small amount of protein in the urine is called *microalbuminuria*, while an excessive amount of protein is termed *macroalbuminuria*. Excessive accumulation of protein in the urine reveals kidney disease, which may lead to end-stage renal disease (ESRD).

Although kidney disease (nephropathy) occurs in diabetes, not everyone is at risk. Precursors to kidney disease in diabetic patients include high blood pressure, heredity, and uncontrolled blood sugar. One may not be aware of their kidney condition in the absence of holistic diagnosis. People occasionally become aware of their condition only when it is too late to save both kidneys, and possibly the entire renal system.

Eye diseases, such as glaucoma, cataracts, and diabetic retinopathy—a disorder of the retina—are another common complication in diabetics. Glaucoma is identified as excessive pressure buildup in the eyeball. The intraocular pressure damages the retina and the optic nerve, which projects from the rear of the eyeball. This eventually leads to blindness. Diabetes also increases the risk of gum disease because of soaring glucose levels.

You can develop nerve damage or diabetic neuropathy regardless of the type of diabetes you have. In diabetic neuropathy, the nerves don't function exactly as they should, causing pain, numbness, weakness, and tingling sensations in the hands and feet. The pain is referred to as *peripheral neuropathy*. The other type of neuropathy is known as *autonomic neuropathy*. In this case, the diabetic patient experiences digestive issues such as nausea, vomiting, diarrhea, and constipation. The bladder malfunctions, and dizziness, fainting, decreased reaction to light and dark surroundings, and loss of libido occur. Other effects include painful feet, skin changes, and emotional instability.

TYPE 1 DIABETES UNCOVERED

Type 1 diabetes occurs when the body stops producing insulin. Following a diagnosis of Type 1 diabetes, you will have to depend on insulin for as long as you live unless a cure for diabetes is discovered sometime in the near future. This is different from Type 2 diabetes, where there is insulin resistance and only moderate insulin deficiency. Type 1 diabetes, as Dr. Peters puts it, "often has a more dramatic start."

Here is a very typical example of someone with Type 1 diabetes: a lanky kid with no family history of diabetes, who is always thirsty, continuously loses weight, and becomes ill very suddenly. When the condition worsens, the child may acquire DKA and should be taken to the hospital as soon as possible. DKA occurs when the body has very limited amounts of insulin, causing acids and ketones to build up unnecessarily.

Beta cells in the pancreas are destroyed in Type 1 diabetes. However, the body seems to get confused, mistaking beta cells for other types of cells, and starts attacking them. The manufactured antibodies mark beta cells and islets of Langerhans for attack, and thus the problem becomes one of auto-immune functioning. A diagnosis of antibodies for islet cells at around six months after the onset of diabetes can signal DKA. Anti-insulin antibodies will also test positive, so for more accuracy, avoid taking insulin shots when taking DKA tests.

In Type 1 diabetes, the beta cells do not die off immediately but rather deteriorate gradually. The process is slow, and when about half the cells are lost, glucose begins to climb. The presence of other illnesses in the body exacerbates insulin resistance. People who have already had their beta cells destroyed—by autoimmune disease, for instance—will be at higher risk.

Diabetics can opt to have their pancreas removed, but this destroys the alpha and beta cells. Alpha cells are responsible for producing the hormone glucagon, the antipode of insulin. Adults who have Type 1 diabetes may fall into the category of latent autoimmune diabetes of the adult (LADA). Just like children who incur Type 1 diabetes, adults who have this illness develop the symptoms gradually. It is sometimes mistaken for Type 2, but, unlike the latter, it involves gradual destruction of the beta cells.

When investigating the possibility of LADA, the blood is tested for anti-glutamic acid decarboxylase (GAD) antibodies. These antibodies affect the levels of gamma-aminobutyric acid (GABA), a chemical needed for healthy muscles. The antibodies linger around for several years, so you should find out from your doctor whether you have LADA.

EASY TRACKING OF TYPE 1 DIABETES

To recognize Type 1 diabetes, keep in mind that those afflicted are usually young and thin, do not have a serious family history of diabetes, and do not belong to any of the following ethnicities: American Indian, African American,

Latino, Asian American, or Pacific Islander. These ethnicities are not known to be at high risk for Type 2 diabetes either.

Insulin is usually administered if the body ceases to respond to medications typically prescribed to diabetics. Type 1 diabetes also affects adults, so if you or your loved ones exhibit the symptoms and have been diagnosed with Type 2 diabetes, it may be wise to seek a second opinion, as the two are so often confused. After being diagnosed, it is advisable to seek a specialist such as an endocrinologist rather than a general practitioner who rarely handles such cases.

Dealing with Type 1 diabetes is all about the interpretation of data and taking notes of sugar levels and insulin doses. Calculating your carbohydrate intake is similarly important. The latest innovations in monitoring and treating this illness need to be utilized.

CONDITIONS ASSOCIATED WITH TYPE 1 DIABETES: CELIAC DISEASE

Type 1 diabetes and celiac disease are perhaps linked to one another. Celiac disease is a digestive disease that damages the linings of the small intestine. The illness later interferes with the absorption of nutrients from food. A person who has this disease cannot tolerate gluten, a protein substance present in wheat, rye, and barley. If we examine someone's medical history and learn that he or she is allergic to wheat and other types of grains, celiac disease is suspected.

For a long time, people with this disease were unaware of this condition because it can begin in childhood. Diarrhea is often a major problem, but not everyone with celiac disease experiences this for the long term.

Signs and symptoms of celiac disease include loss of appetite, weight loss, retardation in children, depression, fatigue, skin rash, anemia, and hypoglycemia, especially for diabetic patients.

According to statistics, one out of twenty diabetic patients has celiac disease. The prevalence of celiac disease in Type 2 diabetics is a lot less at 1 in 250.

Once diagnosed with celiac disease, your diet should exclude all gluten-containing items like bread, crackers, pastas, cookies, and flour. Diabetics with celiac disease generally have a special meal plan laid out for them, but modification may be necessary if other sources of carbohydrates are suspected of interfering with the patient's nutrition. In the end, there will always be alternatives to gluten-containing meals that do not worsen your condition.

You must always watch what you eat, irrespective of whether you have celiac disease. Patients rarely ate restaurant food in the nineteenth century. By the same token, you must only eat foods that you know very well. Find out as much as you can about the ingredients in all the foods you buy.

GESTATIONAL DIABETES: IT NEVER HURTS TO CHECK

In the United States, 3 to 8 percent of pregnant women develop gestational diabetes. Also known as "carbohydrate intolerance of variable severity with onset or first recognition during pregnancy," gestational diabetes was first recognized in 1946. The diagnosis is no different from that of Type 1 and Type 2 diabetes. Many prenatal deaths result from women who develop diabetes during pregnancy, which explains why some experts argue that gestational diabetes is the real third type of diabetes.

Gestational diabetes is attributed to the weight gain and hormonal changes that take place during pregnancy. These are natural phases of pregnancy, but if the changes affect insulin production, then diabetes can soon emerge. In gestational diabetes, the body does not receive the energy it is entitled to because of insulin malfunction.

Predisposing factors for gestational diabetes are similar to those for other types of diabetes: a family history of diabetes, certain ethnicities, age, obesity, a history of gestational diabetes or giving birth to a baby over nine pounds, and prediabetes. As always, remembering these key points can help you prevent gestational diabetes.

The severity of symptoms in gestational diabetes varies immensely among patients. If you think you are at high risk, you should have your blood glucose checked during your first prenatal visit. If the level is ordinary, it should be tested again in the twenty-fourth to twenty-eighth week of pregnancy. If you are at average risk, blood sugar should be screened during the twenty-fourth to twenty-eighth week of pregnancy.

Gestational diabetes tests are usually administered based on risk factors. You may undergo a fasting blood glucose test, a random blood glucose test, a screening glucose challenge test, or an oral glucose tolerance test.

In a fasting blood glucose test, you cannot eat or drink anything for eight hours prior to commencing the test. In a random blood glucose test, the level is checked at any time of the day. These checks are usually enough to determine whether a childbearing woman has diabetes, but if the doctor needs further confirmation, other tests may be performed as well.

The glucose challenge test is performed by drinking a very sweet liquid and then checking sugar levels after an hour. This can be done at any time, and if the results are higher than usual, further testing may be carried out.

For the full glucose tolerance test, you can eat normally for a minimum of three days prior to testing and then fast for eight hours before drinking a very sweet beverage. Your blood glucose level is then checked after one hour, two hours, and three hours. When two out of the three tests come up unusually high, the doctor may diagnose you with gestational diabetes.

By now you are probably wondering what happens to a baby whose mother has gestational diabetes. If left uncontrolled or untreated, the baby is at risk for developing serious complications, like a mismatch between the baby's size and gestational age, low blood sugar, and trouble breathing.

The mother will usually be asymptomatic even if she already has gestational diabetes. This poses a huge risk for high blood pressure and enlargement of the baby if not addressed at the right time. Tests like ultrasounds are therefore ordered to monitor the growth of the fetus. An ultrasound technician keeps tabs on the progress of the baby inside the womb. Special stress tests and kick counts are recorded to determine the baby's activity levels.

You should also have your blood sugar levels checked about six to twelve weeks following delivery. Gestational diabetes goes away after pregnancy if managed well, but it could turn into Type 2 diabetes if left uncontrolled. It may also reoccur during the next pregnancy.

Management of gestational diabetes includes a healthy meal plan, physical activity, and, if necessary, shots of insulin. Because you are carrying a baby at the time, it is recommended that you also consult with a dietitian to learn about the baby's requirements for nutrition and diet.

Having the right diet when you are pregnant will help keep blood glucose levels within a reasonable range. The dietitian can also advise you on the amount of food to eat and the frequency of meals. More or less, you'll be told to restrict sweets, eat three meals with one to three snacks every day, and be mindful of the amount of carbohydrates you eat.

The following discussion describes measures you can take to prevent the reoccurrence of gestational diabetes and the development of Type 2 diabetes.

Keep your weight in proportion to your height and try to stay at your ideal body size. Though your weight is above your ideal body weight (IBW), losing at least 5 to 7 percent of your weight should be a good start. For instance, if you weigh two hundred pounds, losing around ten to fourteen pounds will go a long way toward reducing your chances of developing gestational diabetes.

Physical activity is highly recommended as long as it is done in moderation. Dancing, swimming, or walking for thirty minutes every day can help you avoid gestational diabetes.

Choose meals with grains, vegetables, and fruits. Stay away from high-fat foods and large amounts of calories, and have your blood glucose checked regularly.

Healthy blood glucose levels can be easily achieved through routine walking, swimming, and other simple physical activities. Your health care provider can suggest other, nontraditional activities to keep your blood sugar in check.

If you really need insulin, your health care provider will teach you how to administer this yourself. Giving yourself insulin won't harm the fetus, considering the fact that insulin lacks the ability to travel from your own bloodstream to the baby. Your doctor will train you on how to monitor your sugars using a meter at home. By doing this, you can avoid frequent visits to the clinic or hospital.

THE POSSIBILITY FOR ANOTHER TYPE OF DIABETES

The search for another type of diabetes has been underway ever since doctors discovered that insulin is present in the brain. There is a theory that diabetes may be connected to Alzheimer's disease and may pave the way for additional types of diabetes.

Researchers at Rhode Island Hospital and Brown Medical School found that insulin and the proteins related to it are associated with the part of the brain linked to Alzheimer's disease. They also noted that the growth factors for insulin, found in the brain and the pancreas, are vital to the survival of brain cells and test positive in long-term Alzheimer's patients.

Apparently it has already been shown that insulin resistance is related to neurodegeneration, but there is no specific evidence to back up this theory. Neurodegeneration involves the breakdown of the nervous system's cells, called neurons. Nevertheless, the development of theories linking Alzheimer's to diabetes is still thought provoking.

To investigate the proposed link between insulin and Alzheimer's disease, a specific gene abnormality was studied using laboratory rats. The abnormality leads to diminished insulin signals in the brain. Insulin and insulin-like growth factor (IGF) 1 and 2 are released in the neurons present in various regions of the central nervous system. Inhibited insulin in the brain supposedly leads to Alzheimer's disease, but this abnormal condition does not correspond to Type 1 or Type 2 diabetes. As a result, researchers suspect that this multifaceted issue has its roots in the central nervous system.

Such findings and hypotheses prompted medical experts to examine postmortem tissues from patients with Alzheimer's disease. The researchers discovered abnormal growth factors in the hippocampus, the region of the brain responsible for memory. Unfortunately, these irregularities lead to brain cell death.

A February 2009 Reuters UK news release, reported by Julie Steenhuysen, suggests that insulin plays a role in shielding the brain from the proteins that cause Alzheimer's disease. According to researchers from Northwestern University led by William Klein of GlaxoSmithKline (GSK), the drugs Avandia and Rosiglitazone, recommended for diabetes, are meant to protect the brain from the proteins related to Alzheimer's disease. These drugs supposedly increase a person's sensitivity to insulin. Their conclusion thus far is that Alzheimer's disease is almost like a separate type of diabetes occurring in the brain!

Klein reiterates that in his research he has found that strengthening the signaling of insulin shields the neurons. This study is found in the *Proceedings of the National Academy of Sciences*. In a telephone interview with Reuters, Klein compared the different types of diabetes and mentioned a new type. He pointed out that the pancreas has a difficult time producing insulin in Type 1 patients. In Type 2 patients, the tissues take a hit and become insensitive to insulin due to insulin receptor dilemmas. He went on to list the problems with insulin receptors located in the brain in a new and unresearched form of diabetes.

This condition may take place in old age. As people get older, insulin signaling gets less effective relative to the functioning of the brain. As the brain turns fragile, Alzheimer's disease and other illnesses may occur.

Proteins related to Alzheimer's disease can be traced to "amyloid beta" proteins, which when joined together into large sticky plaques lead to memory loss, confusion, inability to perform the regular activities of daily living, and death. Klein and his colleagues performed studies showing how strands of amyloid beta–derived diffusible ligands (ADDLs) take over the cells of the brain responsible for storing memory. This may introduce memory loss, one of the key diagnostic factors in Alzheimer's. When they tested insulin as a treatment for this condition in rat nerve cells, the results showed that the ADDLs were reversed. Supplementary conclusions were made when rosiglitazone, another drug for diabetes, produced desirable effects on brain function.

Studies also revealed that insulin and IGF 1 are significantly constrained in the frontal cortex, hippocampus, and hypothalamus. All of these parts are also involved in Alzheimer's disease, suggesting that diabetes and Alzheimer's disease may be connected after all. The cerebellum, which is rarely affected by Alzheimer's, did not show any changes and hence supports the overall theory.

Analysts at Mount Sinai Medical Center in New York discovered in 2008 that diabetic patients who take insulin and other diabetes medications are at considerable risk for developing Alzheimer's disease later in life. This study included various types of medications for diabetes, including a class of drugs called sulfonylureas.

In another study conducted in the United States, researchers learned that educating Alzheimer's patients affects the onset and progression of the disease. This could imply that the likelihood of mental deterioration is much greater once you start to lose long-term memory. The findings were based on the results of about 6,500 volunteers.

Furthermore, Robert Wilson, from Rush University Medical Center, published an article suggesting that higher education has no effect on memory loss. As of today, 5.2 million people in the United States are afflicted with Alzheimer's disease, with 26 million worldwide. If you are a diabetic currently suffering from Alzheimer's disease, you should maintain a healthy diet and regular exercise to stave off your physical problems and mental symptoms.

THE FOUR FACES OF DIABETES INSIPIDUS

Our discussion of the types of diabetes would be incomplete without considering diabetes insipidus, abbreviated *DI*. Diabetes insipidus is a specific physical disorder associated with diabetes, be it Type 1 or Type 2. As an obvious and evident symptom of DI, a patient experiences a surprising increase in urine output and a tendency for frequent thirst. DI is generally caused by a lack of vasopressin, a hormone known to control the volume of urine output. There are various indicators by which you can ascertain whether you are suffering from DI. The following list gives a broad scope of DI symptoms:

- Urine quantity increases.
- The patient suffers from nocturia, the habit of waking up in the middle of the night with the urge to urinate. This becomes more frequent as time passes.
- The diabetic patient often exhibits enuresis, or bedwetting. This occurs mostly when the individual is in deep sleep.

Interestingly, DI alters the color of your urine, rendering it very pale and almost colorless. Urine concentration is also distinctly low. Moreover, diabetes insipidus is divided into four major classifications: neurogenic, nephrogenic, dipsogenic, and gestagenic DI.

Neurogenic DI

Neurogenic DI is also known as central, hypothalamic, neurohypophyseal, and pituitary diabetes insipidus. Neurogenic DI involves complications of the nervous system and is the most common form of diabetes insipidus. It is primarily caused by a severe shortage of the hormone vasopressin. Also called antidiuretic hormone (ADH), vasopressin's primary task is to decrease urine volume. ADH also makes the urine highly concentrated.

Nephrogenic DI

The popular name of nephrogenic DI (NDI) is *vasopressin resistant diabetes*. Publications suggest that NDI is mostly brought on by renal (kidney) malfunction. In NDI, the kidneys do not respond adequately to vasopressin. As a result, a person urinates more frequently. NDI patients go through a tremendous amount of suffering because their kidneys fail to conserve water. This is why their urine turns colorless.

Dipsogenic DI

Dipsogenic DI is a special form of diabetes insipidus and is known as a form of primary polydipsia. Dipsogenic DI is characterized by excessive thirst as well. Dipsogenic DI has much in common with neurogenic DI when comparing the symptoms. Dipsogenic DI can be an underlying cause of nausea, lethargy, headache, loss of appetite, and so forth.

Gestagenic DI

Popularly termed in medical circles as *gestational DI*, gestagenic diabetes insipidus is a problem found only in pregnant women. For obvious reasons, pregnant diabetics should always be on the lookout for this special form of diabetes. Gestagenic DI is treated using the medication DDAVP (desmopressin). Symptoms usually fade away after delivery but may reappear in future pregnancies.

Part Two

GETTING TO KNOW DIABETES

· 3 ·

Causes and Symptoms

$\mathcal{D}$o you think that eating too much sugar is the only cause of diabetes? Think again. When exploring the general causes of diabetes, you should note that the symptoms are always somehow related to lifestyle, heredity, and environmental factors. At present, you should know that there are two major types of diabetes: Type 1 and Type 2. In Type 2 diabetes, there are specific factors in question, such as ethnicity, age, obesity, a sedentary lifestyle, pregnancy, and poor diet. In Type 1 diabetes, however, genes and environmental factors play much more important roles.

With advances of technology and the eagerness of medical experts to learn more about diabetes, other causative factors that contribute to this "silent killer" are currently being discovered.

GOING GREEN: ENVIRONMENTAL ASPECTS

In their quest to discover the root cause of Type 1 diabetes, scientists from around the globe worked together to screen 220,800 healthy babies to find any genes that might put them at risk for having Type 1 diabetes. In about four years, they expect to get direct results from 1,300 babies at the very least. Half of the babies will then continue with the study well beyond childhood, hopefully leading researchers to a cure for this dreaded disease.

According to Dr. Jin-Xiong She, professor and director of the Center for Biotechnology and Genomic Medicine at the Medical College of Georgia, the objective is really to determine the environmental factors that lead to Type 1 diabetes. He believes that it is much easier to identify the cure for this disease once you understand the environmental factors responsible.

37

The scientists will monitor almost every detail in the children's everyday life until they come up with theories that provide answers about the environmental contributors to Type 1 diabetes. They will consider every minute detail in the data, such as the water the child drinks, the cookies he or she eats, and many other similar circumstances.

The factors that are suspect include cow's milk containing the Coxsackie virus. This virus is an enterovirus, meaning that it directly affects the intestines. Scientists believe that the Coxsackie virus may have a connection to Type 1 diabetes.

Another ongoing study is The Environmental Determinants of Diabetes in the Young (TEDDY) project. Four states, namely Washington, Georgia, Florida, and Colorado, and three other countries, namely Finland, Sweden, and Germany, joined forces to help out in the project. In the study, families record the diabetic's vitals, including weight, pulse, and blood pressure. They also make note of when the child gets sick, takes medications, goes to a health care provider, and so forth.

Dr. She states that Type 1 diabetes begins in utero, while the baby is still in the womb. This theory, however, has yet to be clinically proven. Project managers are studying the children in the TEDDY project every three months for the first four years and then every six months thereafter until the kids reach the age of fifteen. Although the researchers are only interested in the first fifteen years of the child's life, this does not suggest that the later years are insignificant. The immune system develops in the first years of life, but it continues to evolve throughout life. Noting the health of a Type 1 diabetic during childhood is just as important when the person matures into an adult because it helps determine what to expect with regard to the health of a Type 1 diabetic in his or her later years.

Lack of the mineral zinc in a person's circulation may lay the foundation for diseases like diabetes, cancer, and Alzheimer's. Hypozincemia is a deficiency in zinc that leads to malfunctions of organs and of vital functions such as eyesight, taste, and memory. Hypozincemia may be associated with chronic renal disease, diabetes, and other chronic illnesses. A biomedical imaging sensor is employed by advanced medical facilities to identify zinc levels in the body.

Lack of vitamin D and calcium are also thought to be factors that can initiate diseases like diabetes, multiple sclerosis, malignancies (in the colon, breast, and prostate gland), and other autoimmune and chronic inflammatory disorders.

WE ARE WHO WE WERE: THE GENETICS OF DIABETES

It has been thought for some time that genes are capable of causing diabetes, and medicine has shown this theory to be quite accurate. Researchers have discovered that the gene HLA II, found on chromosome 6p21, is a factor that can cause Type 1 diabetes and celiac disease.

The largest genetic study ever published tells of four chromosome regions with genes associated with Type 1 diabetes and three brand new genes linked to Crohn's disease. The researchers also point out that they have found the gene that connects these two diseases.

Experts believe there are two factors related to both Type 1 and Type 2 diabetes that must be considered. First, there could be a natural predisposition to diabetes. Second, something in the environment must be involved in directly triggering the disease. Though genes alone are not enough to cause diabetes, they do play a major role. Therefore, let's take a detailed look at the genetic causes of Types 1 and 2 diabetes.

Type 1 Diabetes

If Type 1 diabetes develops entirely due to genetics, then both parents of the patient must have diabetes. Type 1 diabetes is more prevalent in Caucasians than in any other ethnicity. According to the American Diabetes Association, if you are a male with Type 1 diabetes, there is a 1 in 17 chance that your child will have this type of diabetes. Meanwhile, if you are a female, the ratio is 1 in 25. If you have a child after the age of twenty-five, the heredity factor is 1 in 100. Having diabetes prior to age eleven also increases the chance that your child will have diabetes.

An estimated one in seven Type 1 diabetics may conjointly have the following conditions: Type 2 polyglandular autoimmune syndrome, thyroid disease, an adrenal gland that does not function well, and other immune disorders. The presence of these conditions amplifies the chance of passing diabetes on to your child to 1 in 2. That is a 50 percent chance of getting diabetes!

Scientists are constantly searching for a system that can help predict the odds of acquiring diabetes. For instance, whites have the genes for HLA-DR3 or HLA-DR4. HLA, or human leukocyte antigens, are foreign material that mediate graft-versus-host disease. If both you and your child bear these genes, and if you are Caucasian, then the risk is higher. For other ethnicities, this field of medicine is currently not very popular, and it would be helpful if experts would spend more time developing such research tools. African Americans have the gene for HLA-DR7, while the Japanese have HLA-DR9.

Cold weather is another factor that researchers are looking into as a cause of Type 1 diabetes. They believe that Type 1 diabetes is more damaging during winter than in summer and has a higher rate of occurrence in places with cooler climates than in those with warmer climates.

Viruses have been a target for researchers who theorize that some viruses that produce mild effects in healthy humans may lead to advanced Type 1 diabetes in others.

A child's upbringing and nourishment may contribute to diabetes to a certain extent. Scientists have found that children who were breast-fed have a decreased risk of suffering from diabetes in later stages of life. Meanwhile, children who were bottle-fed or ate solid foods are more likely to end up with diabetes.

Autoantibodies have a greater chance of being present in diabetic patients even at an early age, making them more susceptible to diabetes later on in life.

Type 2 Diabetes

With Type 2 diabetes, there is a greater genetic contribution, but environmental factors are also being considered.

Once an individual has Type 2 diabetes, he or she can pass it on more easily to family members. Westerners are also at higher risk for this condition because they eat foods with high amounts of fat and low levels of fiber. Since Westerners rely more heavily on technological innovations that discourage physical movement, their lack of exercise contributes to developing diabetes later in life. In the United States, ethnic groups with a greater risk for Type 2 diabetes are Mexican Americans, Pima Indians, and African Americans.

People with habits contrary to those described above have a lower risk of developing Type 2 diabetes, even with a strong family history of the disease. Obesity is also one of the main causes of diabetes. If you recall the pathophysiology of diabetes, fats are broken down, and eventually ketones are produced, causing ketoacidosis. Being overweight doesn't make things any better. It may cause malfunctioning of the pancreas and other organs faster than you think.

Like Type 1 diabetes, the risk for Type 2 can be hereditary. If you have Type 2 diabetes before you turn fifty, the chances of your child inheriting it are 1 in 7. If you are older than fifty when you get diabetes, the chances are 1 in 13.

Experts suggest that if the mother has diabetes, the risk to the child is much more elevated. Diabetes can also affect a developing baby over the entire span of a pregnancy. In early pregnancy, a mother's diabetes can produce birth defects in major organs, such as the brain and heart, and can possibly lead to miscarriage. If both parents have Type 2 diabetes, the risk to the fetus is 1 in 2. Children of parents with varying degrees of Type 2 diabetes also have varied risk factors. In the case of maturity onset diabetes of the young, the risk is 50 percent.

PHYSIOLOGICAL SYMPTOMS IN THE DIABETIC

Blood pressure is one condition currently being investigated with respect to the physiological processes that contribute to diabetes. The chances of getting diabetes are three times greater for women who suffer from increasing or elevated blood pressure levels than for those with regular blood pressure. This result is said to be independent of BMI (body mass index) and other conditions that lead to heart disease and diabetes.

VIRAL FACTORS EXPOSED

Experts suspect that viruses also play a role in the spread of diabetes on a global scale. They say that arsenic, a toxin that makes the body exceptionally vulnerable to viruses like influenza A, disrupts hormone pathways. Since the endocrine system controlling our hormones is one of the most influential body systems we have, hormonal disruption always plays a big role in diseases. Diabetes is a disease of the endocrine system more than anything else.

As of now, the influenza A virus does not appear to have a direct connection to diabetes. Japanese medical experts have discovered that the hepatitis C virus has a direct link to diabetes by way of insulin resistance. Why? As you may know, hepatitis C is a noncancerous liver disease, and insulin is a hormone that permits the conversion of glucose into energy in the liver and muscles. An insulin resistant liver overproduces glucose. Insulin resistant muscles fail to absorb glucose from the bloodstream adequately. In both the liver and the muscles, the end product is a detrimental amount of sugars, which can of course lead to Type 2 diabetes.

CLINICAL MANIFESTATIONS

Signs and symptoms that are common among all types of diabetes are collectively referred to as the "Three Ps":

- Polydipsia—excessive thirst
- Polyuria—excessive urination
- Polyphagia—uncontrolled appetite

Polyuria and polydipsia result from the high levels of fluid lost via osmotic dieresis, the excretion of glucose with water and certain electrolyte molecules through the kidneys. Meanwhile, insulin deficiency causes polyphagia (eating too much), which in turn causes the catabolism (breakdown) of proteins and fats.

Symptoms include abrupt changes in vision, fatigue, weakness, numbness or tingling in the hands and feet, dry skin, wounds that refuse to heal, and various types of infections.

When DKA (diabetic ketoacidosis) has taken over a Type 1 diabetic, the onset is most often marked either by a sudden loss of weight and nausea, or by vomiting sensations and pains in the abdomen.

WHY VISION AND SKIN PROBLEMS OCCUR IN DIABETIC PATIENTS

Diabetic patients often experience blurred vision, dry or itchy skin, and other related conditions. Why does this happen?

Due to high blood sugar levels, fluid is drawn out of the tissues and the lenses of the eyes, which in a roundabout way means that glucose is unable to accumulate in the right places. The extremities of the body, such as the hands and feet, also become dry because of this.

Neuropathy, the tingling sensations already mentioned, occurs when the minor blood vessels that supply blood to the nerves are damaged due to excessive amounts of glucose. Neuropathy manifests itself as fatigue, dehydration due to frequent urination, and the body's inability to convert sugar into energy.

Skin infections and wounds that refuse to heal develop as a result of a weakened immune system, which allows deadly microorganisms to invade the body.

OTHER MILD SYMPTOMS

Milder symptoms that accompany diabetes include abscesses, athlete's foot, urinary tract infections, candida, thrush, flaky skin, skin ulcers, drowsiness, and other skin infections. As a safety measure, detailed knowledge of preventative measures and an ability to recognize these mild symptoms helps in the struggle against diabetes.

Mild weight loss due to diabetes is attributed to the loss of nutrients and minerals as they are passed out through the urine. As a result of having diabetes, sugar may not reach the cells, thereby contributing to excessive hunger. When this happens, Type 1 diabetes occurs almost naturally.

Athlete's Foot

Athlete's foot, as a mild symptom of diabetes, is a type of skin disorder caused by a fungus. The medical name of this particular fungus is *Trichophyton*. Another organism assumed to have ties to athlete's foot is ringworm, medically identified as *tinea*. The most alarming characteristic of ringworm is that it usually makes its home in lower regions like the legs, but it can also ascend to other parts of the body, including the hands, groin, and nails.

If you ever suspect athlete's foot, you need to look for serious warning signs. Irritation at the edge of your feet does not warrant an official diagnosis of athlete's foot. An individual suffering from athlete's foot is likely to exhibit specific signs. The patient's feet might have a reddish look, and dry skin would be noticeable on both soles of the feet. Occasional dry flakes that spread all over the feet are also symptoms of athlete's foot. The patient might also suffer from the presence of too much moisture in the feet and peeling skin. That is why it is essential to remove the slightest trace of any fungus or rash sprouting over the toes or any other region.

Brain Abscess

Abscesses are considered one of the harbingers of diabetes. Doctors talk about different types of abscesses, but brain abscesses are rarely on their list. A brain abscess is a pivotal point of discussion in medical science, and it is suggested that brain abscesses affect women more often than men. This special type of abscess can be deep inside the brain, causing the patient physical and emotional concerns.

The inconveniences caused by a brain abscess can include headaches, stuffy nose, bilateral eyeball soreness, low-grade fever, and rhinorrhea (runny nose).

Primary Pituitary Abscess

A primary pituitary abscess is a rare event in the pituitary gland of a human being, regardless of whether the patient is a diabetic. This type of abscess is closely linked to diabetes insipidus. Medical practitioners and researchers observe that this physical disorder usually targets the brain at a very young age. A primary pituitary abscess can be a fatal outcome of a pituitary infection.

The pituitary gland is a hidden gland in the brain that secrets essential hormones. The clinical symptoms pertaining to this physical ailment are fairly atypical and difficult to diagnose. A diabetic who presents the symptoms of a primary pituitary abscess might also have diabetes insipidus syndrome. With this in mind, proper care should be taken after carrying out a thorough diagnosis on the patient.

Dental Abscess

A dental abscess is another pesky type of abscess that tends to come and go. It is an infection of the mouth that affects the face, jaw, and other structures and that weakens the immune system of the human body. Dental abscesses are a mild symptom of diabetes, though medical practitioners theorize that they can also be a direct result of physical trauma.

Sleep Hyperhidrosis

Sleep hyperhidrosis is considered a mild side-effect of diabetes. Sleep hyperhidrosis, also known as nocturnal hyperhidrosis, or night sweating, is a physical disorder that affects diabetics mostly at night. Generally speaking, night sweating doesn't pose a great threat to the patient, but it can be a problem when it is chronic.

This unrelenting form of perspiration takes place only during sleep and disappears when a person is awake. A healthy, fit person pumps out between five hundred and one thousand milliliters of sweat per day, but a diabetic suffering from sleep hyperhidrosis is sure to produce much more.

The Truth about Candidiasis

Candidiasis is one of the most serious and prominent symptoms of diabetes. However, there are several myths associated with its link to diabetes. Candidiasis is a kind of scaly rash that itches. The infection originates from a fungus called *Candida albicans*. If you suspect candidiasis, remember that it tends to occur mostly in the moist and warm areas of the body.

Inflammation, irritation, and itching—these are grounds for a diagnosis of candidiasis, which is yet another serious warning sign in diabetes. Candidiasis feeds on excess blood sugar levels, and after attacking you, it weakens your immune system and makes you more vulnerable to other infections. From a holistic standpoint, the body cannot produce the required amount of insulin, which is an essential element for preventing diabetes if the immune system is weakened. Candidiasis thereby makes sugar levels edge up to an alarming level. In order to treat this condition, your doctor may prescribe a generic antifungal cream such as ketoconazole or miconazole. These medications work great on just about any kind of fungus, even on molds and yeasts.

Note that chronic symptoms of candidiasis may be a sign of impending diabetes, but proper treatment and management can keep candidiasis and diabetes at bay.

LATER SYMPTOMS

As the sugar level rises, symptoms also increase in severity. Aside from the Three Ps, the following symptoms may also occur:

- Muscle aches
- Cramps
- Headaches
- Irritability
- Erectile dysfunction
- Vaginal dryness
- Absent menstrual periods
- Acne that worsens or improves depending on high or low sugar levels

ACUTE COMPLICATIONS IN DIABETIC PATIENTS

Three major complications pertain to diabetes in the short term: hypoglycemia, DKA, and hyperglycemic hyperosmolar syndrome.

Hypoglycemia

An abnormally low blood sugar level occurs when the level falls between 50 and 60 mg/dL, or between 2.7 and 3.3 mmol/L. This might be the result of high amounts of insulin, oral hypoglycemic medications, very little food, or certain physical activities. Hypoglycemia can occur at any time throughout the day but occurs most often after going a long time without eating anything. Midmorning hypoglycemia, for example, strikes on those mornings when you have the most insulin in you. Typical hypoglycemia creeps up in the late afternoon and follows its midmorning counterpart. If you don't eat anything before bedtime, midnight hypoglycemia can occur.

General hypoglycemia can be classified into two categories based on the type of symptoms: adrenergic symptoms and central nervous system (CNS) symptoms.

There are instances in which the response time of hormones, also known as the adrenergic response, is diminished. This may be linked to autonomic neuropathy, which is a chronic or long-term complication. During such instances, the usual flow of adrenalin is absent, and the person does not experience the common adrenergic symptoms like shakiness and sweating. Hypoglycemia is not imminent unless moderate or severe symptoms occur.

Mild fluctuations in blood sugar stimulate the sympathetic nervous system to call for an excess flow of the hormones epinephrine and norepinephrine. Symptoms like sweating, tachycardia (higher than normal heart rate), tremors, palpitations, hunger, and nervousness can then occur.

In moderate hypoglycemia, the brain cells do not receive the glucose needed to function well, thus evoking the following:

- Light-headedness
- Headache
- Memory lapses
- Confusion
- Numbness of the lips and tongue
- Impaired coordination
- Slurred speech
- Irrational or combative behavior
- Shifts in emotions
- Double vision
- Drowsiness

A combination of these symptoms can occur in the presence of adrenergic abnormalities that caused the mild hypoglycemia in the first place.

In severe hypoglycemia, there is major malfunctioning of the CNS that brings about seizures, disorientation, difficulty waking up, and even loss of consciousness.

All of these symptoms may occur unexpectedly and can vary depending on the mental and physical state of the person. For instance, you could experience these symptoms if your sugar levels drop from 200 to 120 mg/dL, especially if you are used to having irregular sugar levels. On the contrary, when an individual is almost always hypoglycemic, more often than not there are no symptoms involved.

ENTER, DIABETIC KETOACIDOSIS

We have mentioned diabetic ketoacidosis (DKA) in previous chapters, but this time we will go into more detail.

Diabetic ketoacidosis is one of the more notorious complications of diabetes. It is mainly caused by inadequate levels of insulin. As a DKA patient, you may be unable to properly metabolize lipids, carbohydrates, and proteins. When DKA attacks, three noteworthy symptoms follow: hyperglycemia, dehydration and electrolyte loss, and acidosis.

Malfunctions of insulin cause glucose to enter the liver and muscles at a minimal rate. Subsequently, the liver compensates by increasing the amount of glucose it manufactures. This reaction brings on hyperglycemia. Then the body tries to get rid of the extra glucose by excreting glucose with water and electrolytes (e.g., sodium and potassium) via the kidneys.

This process is called osmotic diuresis, which is also responsible for polyuria, dehydration, and loss of electrolytes. When there is severe dehydration involved, there may be a loss of 6.5 liters of water and 400 to 500 mEq, or milliequivalent, for sodium, chloride, and potassium within a short amount of time.

Osmotic diuresis leads to the breakdown of fat, a process known as lipolysis, into glycerol and free fatty acids. Over time, the liver turns these free fatty acids to ketones. Ketones then enter the bloodstream and pass into the circulation just like any other organic molecule, but in this case leading to metabolic acidosis.

The causes of DKA have been traced to failure to use insulin, an illness or infection, and diabetes that for some reason has gone unreported.

The symptoms of DKA include polyuria, polydipsia, blurred vision, headache, and weakness. A stark decrease of 20 mmHg or more in systolic blood pressure upon standing may indicate orthostatic hypotension. When you have this form of hypotension, your blood pressure falls as you stand up. A weak, rapid pulse immediately follows. Normally the opposite effect occurs; the blood pressure of a person standing up intensifies to allow nutrients to flow into the brain.

Ketosis and acidosis from DKA cause gastrointestinal symptoms like anorexia, nausea, vomiting, and abdominal pain. Due to the high levels of ketone, your breath will have a fruity odor to it, similar to that of acetone. There may also be hyperventilation, with respirations that are deep but not labored. Kussmaul breathing, which involves deep and labored respirations, is a form of hyperventilation that indicates you are trying to fight acidosis and the buildup of ketones.

The mental states involved in DKA may vary. A certain number of patients may be either alert, lethargic, or comatose depending on plasma osmolarity. Plasma osmolarity indicates how hydrated a person is.

Hyperglycemic Hyperosmolar Nonketotic Syndrome (HHNS)

This condition is a combination of hyperosmolarity and hyperglycemia. It is distinguished by an altered sense of awareness or a lack of sensorium. Sensorium refers to an individual's sensation, perception, and interpretation of the surrounding environment.

As a result of ongoing hyperglycemia, osmotic diuresis (increased urination) occurs and leads to water and electrolyte loss. To maintain a stable osmotic process, water travels from the fluid inside cells to the fluid space outside of the cell. Owing mostly to dehydration and glucosuria, sodium levels become extremely high. This lays the foundation for unwanted hypernatremia (too much sodium).

Older individuals aged fifty to seventy often have HHNS. Nondiabetics are just as prone to this condition as diabetics and those with mild Type 2 diabetes are. According to various studies, the root cause may be due to having an acute disease such as stroke or pneumonia, taking medications that aggravate hyperglycemia like thiazides, or dialysis treatment procedures.

Victims of HHNS generally experience polyuria, or frequent urination, in the preliminary stages of the disease. HHNS differs from DKA because the former does not involve any ketosis or acidosis. There are also varying levels of insulin in HHNS. However, in DKA, sufficient insulin is not there, so glucose, protein, and stored fat start to break down. Sadly, this produces ketones and consequently ketoacidosis.

Hyperglycemia and osmotic dieresis are both expected to occur in HHNS because of the low levels of insulin. Meanwhile, if the insulin level shoots up, you won't be able to metabolize or break down any fats.

There are no gastrointestinal symptoms related to ketosis that would prompt an HHNS patient to seek treatment. In most cases they can still handle polyuria and polydipsia unless there are neurological changes or illnesses that have grave effects. Due to the delay in treatment, dehydration, hyperglycemia, and hyperosmolarity turn out to be more severe in HHNS than in DKA.

The following clinical manifestations are frequently signs of HHNS:

- Dry mucous membranes and poor skin turgor
- Tachycardia, or rapid pulse
- Hypotension, or low blood pressure
- Significant dehydration
- Varying neurological signs such as alteration of the senses, seizures, and hemiparesis (weakness on only one side of the body)

The mortality rate of HHNS is 10 to 40 percent, with roots to other chronic illnesses and complications, which we will discuss later.

CHRONIC COMPLICATIONS: WHEN THE WRECKING BALL JUST KEEPS GOING

Besides acute complications, there are chronic manifestations related to the cardiovascular system and the renal system which, together with other conditions, inhibit a diabetic from performing activities of daily living (ADLs).

Today, more and more people are suffering from complications that fall into three categories: macrovascular disease, microvascular disease, and neuropathy.

Physical processes that lead to these complications are being studied, and experts believe that abnormal levels of blood glucose bring about neuropathic illnesses, microvascular complications, and risk factors that lead to other major difficulties. They also believe that high blood pressure plays an important role in macrovascular and microvascular disease. Long-term issues may occur in both Type 1 and Type 2 diabetes, but these reactions develop about five to ten years after the initial diagnosis. They may be present at the time of the diagnosis of Type 2 diabetes but remain unnoticeable for a while, which is why diabetes is referred to as the silent killer. Type 2 diabetes goes undiagnosed every now and then unless grave symptoms occur.

Renal and microvascular disorders usually affect people with Type 1 diabetes, whereas cardiovascular (macrovascular) disease is found more often with Type 2 diabetes.

MACROVASCULAR COMPLICATIONS

Changes take place in medium and large blood vessels. The walls of the blood vessels develop plaque, which ultimately restricts the flow of blood. If these complications are related to diabetes, they are observed at an earlier age. Three main types of macrovascular disease affect diabetics: cerebrovascular disease (brain dysfunctions), coronary artery disease (heart disease), and peripheral vascular disease (the obstruction of large arteries in the arms and legs).

Myocardial infarctions, commonly referred to as *heart attacks*, are also often observed in diabetics. With today's sedentary lifestyle, people are more prone to this illness. It is twice as common in men with diabetes and three times as common in women with the disease.

Once afflicted with myocardial infarction, the possibility of having other complications increases, as does the chance for a second attack.

Of the deaths caused by diabetes, around 50 to 60 percent are the result of coronary artery disease. Therefore it is important to learn about the symptoms and underlying pathological agents that cause this incapacitating illness.

In coronary artery disease related to diabetes, the usual ischemic symptoms are absent. You may not have reduced coronary blood flow, thus causing "silent" myocardial infarctions. To detect virtually any heart disease, you have to undergo an electrocardiogram (EKG) test. The cause of nutrient-starving heart symptoms can be traced to autonomic neuropathy, which is discussed below.

Progressing atherosclerosis affects the cerebral blood vessels, which could end up with an occlusion. Changes in the occlusion may form a clot (embolus) that blocks smaller vessels and produces transient ischemic attacks and strokes.

Diabetics have a greater risk of developing cerebrovascular disease that ends in death. With elevated blood glucose levels, the chances of recovering from a stroke are minimal. Due to the similarity between cerebrovascular disease and acute diabetic complications such as HHNS or hypoglycemia, glucose levels need to be tested and managed as soon as these symptoms are noticed to prevent further injury.

Moreover, occlusive peripheral arterial diseases (PADs) are usually brought on by changes that are atherosclerotic in nature. PAD occurs a lot in the large vessels of the lower extremities. In peripheral vascular disease, the pulses of the lower limbs are virtually nonexistent, and related intermittent claudication (clotting) produces severe pain in the buttock, thigh, or calf while walking. Once the arterial occlusive disease in the lower extremities becomes severe, gangrene (decay of body tissues) sets in, and in certain cases amputation takes place. In diabetic foot diseases, neuropathy and prolonged wound healing are the major concerns.

MICROVASCULAR COMPLICATIONS

Microvascular injuries are possible in all types of diabetes. In diabetic microvascular disease, or microangiopathy, the capillary basement membrane thickens, creating a blockage of the endothelial capillary cells. There are basic biochemical responses related to high blood glucose levels that lead to thickening of the membrane. Due to these changes, the retinas of the eyes and the kidneys are also affected.

Let us look now to diabetic retinopathy, the leading cause of vision impairment in American diabetics aged twenty to seventy-four. Diabetic retinopathy affects both Type 1 and Type 2 diabetes patients. One out of every four patients undergoing kidney dialysis suffers from diabetic retinopathy.

Diabetic patients are prone to numerous visual complications. This condition, referred to as diabetic retinopathy, involves harmful changes in the small blood vessels located in the retina, the part of the eye that receives images and transmits them to the brain. Various blood vessels, like small arteries and veins, venules, arterioles, and capillaries, fill the retina. Three main stages are present in diabetic retinopathy: nonproliferative (background) retinopathy, preproliferative retinopathy, and proliferative retinopathy.

Almost all Type 1 diabetics and about 60 percent of those with Type 2 diabetes will have some amount of visual difficulty within twenty years of getting diabetes. Changes in microvasculature include intraretinal hemorrhages, microaneurysms, focal capillary closure, and hard exudates.

Though most patients do not develop visual impairment, it can be devastating when it does occur. Nonproliferative retinopathy and macular edema develop in 10 percent of people with Type 1 and Type 2 diabetes. This may lead to distortion of vision and central vision loss.

An advanced form of background retinopathy, known as preproliferative retinopathy, serves as a precursor to a much riskier condition called proliferative retinopathy. In this condition, vascular changes are more extensive, and nerve fibers are eventually lost. Between 10 to 50 percent of people with preproliferative retinopathy are expected to develop proliferative retinopathy in a short time, one year at the most. Furthermore, macular edema is closely linked to preproliferative retinopathy.

Proliferative retinopathy is among the most dangerous threats to vision and is indicated by a spread of new blood vessels growing from the retina to the vitreous. These new vessels have a tendency to bleed, and therefore loss of vision related to proliferative retinopathy is caused by hemorrhaging in the vitreous or retinal detachment.

The vitreous is supposed to be clear so that light can be transmitted to the retina. Once there is hemorrhaging, the vitreous becomes clouded and cannot transmit light, leading to loss of vision. Aside from the vitreous hemorrhage, there is massive scar tissue formation due to the reabsorption of fluid in the eye vessels. This causes vitreous B predicaments on the retina and precedes retinal detachment and later vision impairment.

Retinopathy may or may not be painful. After macular edema, blurry vision occurs both in preproliferative and nonproliferative retinopathy. However, many patients turn out to be asymptomatic, meaning they lack any visible warning signs. Diabetics with a substantial degree of proliferative retinopathy and some hemorrhaging may not suffer from vision loss at all. They should be on the lookout for floaters within their visual field, as well as sudden minor visual changes.

GIVE YOUR KIDNEYS A CHANCE: NEPHROPATHY AND DIABETES

Another common complication of diabetes is renal disease, or nephropathy, caused by diabetic microvascular changes in the kidneys. Long-term diabetics contribute to about half of the new cases of end-stage renal disease (ESRD) every single year. Approximately one out of four ESRD diabetics receives dialysis or undergoes a kidney transplant in the United States. Around 20 to 30 percent of those with Type 1 or Type 2 diabetes soon have nephropathy. There are many more Type 1 patients with ESRD than Type 2 patients. African Americans, Hispanics, and Native Americans with Type 2 diabetes are more prone to ESRD than Caucasians.

Once you have diabetes, the capacity of the kidneys to filter the blood is stressed, causing blood proteins to leak into the urine. The pressure on the blood vessels in the kidneys then peaks. Experts now conclude that nephropathy occurs because of the elevated blood pressure. Nowadays, different medications and diets are being developed and tested to prevent the development of such complications.

The usual signs and symptoms of renal dysfunction in diabetic patients are the same for nondiabetics. As renal failure occurs, the breakdown (catabolism) of exogenous and endogenous insulin slows, thus producing frequent episodes of hypoglycemia. Because of the changes in diet prescribed to people with nephropathy and changes in the breakdown of insulin, growth hormone secretions and insulin production are altered. The stress brought on by renal disease may prompt a reduction in self-esteem and disrupt family connections and marital relations. It can also contribute to multisystem abnormalities like declining visual acuity, foot ulcerations, impotence, nocturnal diarrhea, and heart failure.

NEUROPATHY: PROBLEMS WITH THE NERVES

When the different types of nerves are affected by diabetes and develop into complications, diabetic neuropathy, or nerve pain, begins to form. The peripheral, autonomic, and spinal nerves may be involved. With varying manifestations, this can arise in different nerve cells. The prevalence of diabetic neuropathy depends on the patient's age and the length of time he or she has been a diabetic. The incidence rate may be as high as 50 percent in people who have had diabetes for twenty-five years or more.

Neuropathy is linked to vascular and metabolic processes. Experts believe there may be a thickening of the capillary basement membrane and demyelination of nerves. Interestingly, this is associated with hyperglycemia. When there are issues with the myelin sheaths, the conduction of nerves is interrupted.

The two most typical forms of neuropathy are sensorimotor polyneuropathy and autonomic neuropathy. Elderly individuals may also be inflicted with cranial mononeuropathies, which are dysfunctions of the cranial nerves.

Sensorimotor Polyneuropathy

In sensorimotor polyneuropathy, the distal parts of the nerves, especially those in the lower extremities, are targeted with pain. Both sides of the body are equally affected, and the pain will most likely spread toward the center of the body, suggesting a "proximal" tendency of the disease.

Autonomic Neuropathies

Autonomic neuropathy (AN) is another type of neuropathy that is related to the autonomic nervous system. This disease causes imbalances in almost all organs. It affects the cardiac, renal, and gastrointestinal (GI) systems. In reference to heart symptoms, autonomic neuropathies include slight tachycardia, or fast heart rate, and orthostatic hypotension. Orthostatic hypotension is basically reduced blood pressure due to a quick change in stance or position. Silent, or painless, myocardial ischemia and infarction may also surface from autonomic neuropathies. Other symptoms are emesis (vomiting), bloating, and delayed gastric emptying. Wide swings in sugar levels may occur on short notice due to frequent changes in the absorption of glucose from the foods being eaten. This can cause constipation or diarrhea.

Autonomic neuropathy of the adrenal medulla produces a decrease in or even a total absence of adrenergic symptoms due to hypoglycemia. The adrenal medulla is the middle part of the adrenal gland, which sits atop the kidneys. Victims of autonomic neuropathy may not even display any conspicuous symptoms. This is why it is necessary to take note of the signs and symptoms of hypoglycemia, just to be safe. You never know; you might be suffering from autonomic neuropathy without even noticing.

Peripheral Neuropathy

The earliest symptoms of peripheral neuropathy are tingling and mild burning sensations that can occur just about anywhere. These symptoms are experienced mostly at night. When the condition gets much more serious, the following indicators appear:

- Numbness of the feet
- Decreased recognition of posture

- Inability to determine the position and movement of the body (proprioception)

The above symptoms can cause unsteady gait or poor balance, so it is vital to watch where you are going at all times. Insensitivity to pain and temperature puts you at a high risk for foot injuries and infections.

Individuals with peripheral neuropathy are prone to developing foot deformities and changes in the joints, such as the Charcot joints (joints of the feet). These deformities are caused by an abnormal sense of touch rather than by irregular weight distribution.

With peripheral neuropathy, a person tends to have smaller deep tendon reflexes, so doing a knee-jerk test is probably the best way to see how severe the situation really is. In fact, these reflexes may serve as the only way to identify this complication. It is also important to note additional contributing factors, such as alcohol consumption or vitamin deficiency.

Sudomotor Neuropathy

Sudomotor neuropathy is related to a decrease or absence of sweating (anhidrosis) in the extremities and upper regions of the body. Feet may get excessively dry, which can trigger the possibility of foot ulcers.

Sexual Dysfunction

Autonomic neuropathy leads to sexual dysfunction in men, but research on sexual dysfunction in diabetic females is still in its initial stage. Some studies, however, specify that autonomic neuropathy can lead to vaginal dryness or infection, decreased libido, and vaginal itching. Urinary tract infections and vaginitis may likewise occur.

Diabetic men tend to be impotent (unable to maintain an erection). Besides diabetes, sexual impotence can also be a consequence of antihypertensive medications, psychological issues, or other medical situations like insufficient fluids.

THE MILE RUN: PROBLEMS IN THE FOOT AND LEG

As mentioned before, the loss of sensation in the lower extremities can lead to amputation. In order to combat this, we have to equip ourselves with knowledge regarding the conditions that occur before such a dreadful event takes place.

It starts with an injury to the soft tissues of the foot, the development of fissures between the toes or on any dry area of the skin, or a callus formation. You don't usually feel these injuries, but your foot develops a loss of touch and temperature sensation due to a variety of factors. These include using heating pads, walking barefoot on concrete, or testing bath water using your foot. There may even be physical irritations that occur while cutting nails, removing calluses and corns, or wearing unfitted garments like socks.

MORE INSIGHT ON THE CAUSES OF DIABETES

The antibody known as CTLA-4 is responsible for the maintenance and induction of T-cell tolerance. When it polymorphs (changes) in human cells, autoimmune diseases, such as Type 1 diabetes and thyroid disease may appear.

Researchers at the University of Otago discovered the gene named PTPN22, a rheumatoid hereditary factor linked to Type 1 diabetes and thyroiditis.

According to a project involving 658 multiple sclerosis (MS) victims, people inflicted with MS are highly susceptible to Type 1 diabetes.

Another study involving the development of white blood cells suggests that a defective apoptosis, in which cells experience faulty programming of cell death, can end up changing the entire structure of a cell. Once this occurs, the body goes into autoimmune mode and starts destroying itself gradually.

Read on to chapter 4 to learn about diagnosing Type 1 diabetes, which is heavily associated with autoimmune disease.

• 4 •

Diagnosing Diabetes

$\mathcal{T}$o diagnose prediabetes or diabetes, your primary physician can perform a simple blood test. The fasting blood sugar level is determined, and a full lipid panel is conducted on the patient. The lipid panel analyzes the levels of good and bad cholesterol and triglycerides.

Your blood sugar level can be tested for free at health fairs and other similar events, but for more accurate results, you should have it done at a doctor's office. It may be a good idea to compile the numbers and take note of any big changes in your condition, because that way you're really keeping tabs on the disease. There are three categories of fasting blood glucose levels: a level more than 125 mg/dL designates diabetes. At 100 to 125 mg/dL, you have prediabetes, which puts you at risk for diabetes and heart ailments. A value of less than 100 mg/dL is considered ordinary, but you may still be at risk for heart conditions.

Today, doctors recommend the oral glucose tolerance test over the intravenous glucose tolerance test because of the potential for infection and other general risks associated with pricking your veins. The values of plasma glucose may be 10 to 15 percent greater than whole blood values, which are obtained through finger sticks in the intravenous method. Besides the procedures that are used to assess and diagnose diabetes, there are continual screenings for those who have had the disease for a long time and to search for complications in newly diagnosed patients.

Aging may be one cause of heightened glucose levels. Diabetics experience elevated blood glucose levels during their fifties, and as they get older, it rises. Once we separate diabetics with very noticeable symptoms from the statistics, we see that 10 to 30 percent of the elderly suffer from age-related hyperglycemia. Studies of carbohydrate metabolism and its connection to aging are ongoing. Being overweight, having poor dietary habits, and not engaging in physical activity leads to the storage of fats and to insulin resistance.

A CLOSER LOOK AT MONITORING GLUCOSE LEVELS AND KETONES

To deal with diabetes, strict monitoring of blood glucose levels is required. This is something you can do on your own. The patient who performs self-monitoring of blood glucose (SMBG) is in control of his or her own health and can help with the delivery of timely care.

SMBG allows the detection of hyperglycemia and hypoglycemia so that the patient can seek treatment and prevent complications. The most common method used in SMBG is the blood glucose meter, which reads the level of glucose from a strip with a drop of blood from the fingertip. To obtain a reading, the blood has to stay on the strip for a specific length of time as instructed by the manufacturer (commonly five to thirty seconds).

A whole host of features and technologies come with today's sugar meters. In the newer glucose monitors, one end of the strip is placed into the meter before applying blood to it, and it stays there for the entire length of the test. The meter will give the sugar count in less than one minute.

Some meters act as biosensors that detect blood coming from other test sites, like the forearm. There are specialized lancing devices used in this case, instead of the painful finger sticks.

In addition, meters are available for visually impaired patients. They feature an audio component that guides the patient in performing the test and allows the patient to obtain data with ease. There are also meters that check your sugar amounts *and* ketone levels. These instruments are recommended for patients who are prone to developing diabetic ketoacidosis (caused by high amounts of ketones).

Pros and Cons of SMBG Systems

The right method for obtaining SMBG levels is really determined by the current situation of the diabetic. Factors such as fine motor coordination, visual acuity, cognitive ability, comfort in performing the procedure, willingness, and cost are all factors to be considered.

The least expensive methods are those that are visual and require less equipment. However, the patient must be able to distinguish colors, have the right timing in performing the test, and be able to interpret the results.

Personal meters can be costly these days, and they depend less on technique and more on the willingness to improve. Yet these machines provide far more precise results. If you don't have the budget for such meters, a health care professional can suggest one that is right for you.

The older meters that require removal of the blood from the reagent strip are not used as much today. They require procedures with more steps to follow in sequence. The newer meters do not require that blood be removed and are easier to use.

If you follow the steps incorrectly when checking your sugars, you may end up with errors in your sugar values. Deviations from the correct procedure can include improper application of the specimen, a meter that has not been maintained properly, damage to the reagent strips due to heat or humidity, and use of outdated strips.

The patient must be well educated in employing these devices and should purchase them from suppliers who offer training in the procedures. Every six to twelve months, patients should also have their blood glucose level tested in a laboratory to compare the results with the ones they get from the SMBG. Meter accuracy is best when a new vial is used and if the readings are confirmed by lab test.

Who May Do SMBG?

All diabetics can benefit from SMBG, since it allows patients to care for themselves somewhat. Anyone undergoing intensive insulin therapy, like patients who take two to four injections a day, diabetics who use insulin pumps, and those who have gestational diabetes, are all good candidates for SMBG. SMBG is recommended for people with unstable diabetes, patients who have severe ketosis or high levels of blood glucose, and those who have hypoglycemia without any warning symptoms. Practice self-monitoring whenever you are able.

SMBG is a reliable way of finding out whether the exercise, diet, and oral antidiabetic agents are sufficient for a particular diabetic. You will be much more motivated to pursue a specific form of treatment if the procedures are known to be effective. Self-monitoring is highly recommended when you suspect hyperglycemia or hypoglycemia.

The Frequency of SMBG

For patients on insulin, the recommended SMBG rate is two to four times a day, with one of the tests taken at bedtime. On the other hand, diabetics who are not on insulin should check their blood sugar levels two to three times a week, including a two-hour postprandial (after a meal) test. For all diabetics, SMBG is recommended whenever hyperglycemia or hypoglycemia is imminent. There should also be an evident increase in the frequency of this procedure when there are changes in medications, activity, or diet, and during times of illness or stress.

How to Read the Results of SMBG

To detect specific personal patterns, patients who do SMBG should keep a record of their blood glucose levels. The test can be conducted during the medication's peak effectiveness time to determine if the dosage really needs adjusting. Evaluation of basal insulin for determining the bolus insulin dose can be done prior to meals. A bolus insulin dose is a dose of rapid-acting or regular insulin that is given to a diabetic to cover the food eaten during one sitting. Tests should be performed two hours after eating to try to find the ideal bolus insulin dose.

Type 2 diabetics are advised to take the test before and two hours after the biggest meal of the day, which is usually lunch or dinner. For those who take insulin at bedtime or use an insulin infusion pump, the test should be done at 3 a.m. once a week to ensure that the blood sugar level is not dropping at night. If a person cannot comply with such testing or has insufficient funds, it can be done once or twice a day (for instance, before breakfast on one day and before lunch the next day).

BAD-TASTING GLUCOSE TESTS

Thus far we have discussed SMBG, but we will now deal with the glucose tests used in hospitals and other health care facilities.

The Fasting Plasma Glucose Test

The fasting plasma glucose (FPG) test is done after eight hours of fasting. It is a favorable method for diagnosing diabetes and prediabetes because of its low cost and convenience. It is best to take the FPG test in the morning. People with a fasting glucose level of 100 to 125 mg/dL have prediabetes, or impaired fasting glucose (IFG), and are at risk for Type 2 diabetes. You have Type 2 diabetes when your FPG is 126 mg/dL or higher.

Oral Glucose Tolerance Test

In the oral glucose tolerance test (OGTT), blood glucose is tested eight hours after the patient has eaten and two hours after he or she has drunk a beverage containing about seventy-five grams of glucose. This test is also helpful for diagnosing diabetes and prediabetes.

According to some studies, the OGTT is more accurate than the FPG test, but it is not as convenient to administer. If sugar results are 140 to 199 mg/dL two hours after drinking the beverage, you have impaired glucose tolerance (IGT). Just as with IFG, in patients with IGT there is a heightened chance of developing Type 2 diabetes. Patients who measure more than 200 mg/dL two hours after drinking the sweet beverage on two consecutive days are positive for Type 2 diabetes.

The OGTT is used to test for gestational diabetes, the type of diabetes acquired during pregnancy, through the collected plasma. The liquid for this test, again, contains a hefty seventy-five grams of glucose. Unlike FPG tests, sugar levels are observed four times with OGTT. If the results are elevated on at least two occasions, the woman has gestational diabetes.

Random Plasma Glucose Test

Total sugar levels can be measured any time of the day when you do a random plasma glucose test. Symptoms that have been discussed previously, such as excessive urination and thirst and unexplained weight loss, can be checked with this test.

GLYCOSYLATED HEMOGLOBIN

Also referred to as $HgbA_{1c}$ or A1C, glycosylated hemoglobin refers to a blood test that determines the average blood sugar level over a period of two to three months. If the test result is high, it validates the presence of glucose molecules in the hemoglobin of the red blood cell. Glucose also tends to attach to red cells after hanging around for a while. Glycosylated hemoglobin levels turn out to be higher when glucose remains in circulation as well.

The hemoglobin that has glucose attached to it stays inside the body for as long as the red blood cell lives, which is about four months. If glucose levels are close to the average human values, with only a few fluctuations here and there, then total sugar amounts will not be so bad. However, when total sugar levels are high, so are A1C levels.

If you find your SMBG results to be satisfactory but your glycosylated hemoglobin numbers are abnormal, you may have made an error during your tests. Mistakes can happen due to manual errors or malfunctioning instruments.

Different tests that check the same things may have different names that include hemoglobin A$_{1c}$ and hemoglobin A1. The typical values differ slightly in these tests in different laboratories, but they usually range from 4 to 6 percent. Values near the typical range suggest near normal blood sugar levels.

URINE TESTING FOR THE PRESENCE OF GLUCOSE

Prior to the utilization of SMBG methods, the means used to test for the presence of glucose every day was urine glucose testing. However, this type of test is only for those who cannot or will not perform SMBG. Urine glucose testing has its advantages. It is less expensive and is hardly as invasive as SMBG testing methods. As part of the general process for urine testing, you put urine on a reagent strip or tablet, and then, after waiting a little while, you match the colors on the strip to a color chart.

The results from urine glucose testing may not be accurate enough to determine the level of total glucose. Glucose that bypasses the kidneys and ends up in the urine is known as the glucose renal threshold. If the renal threshold is at a level of 180 to 200 mg/dL, or 9.9 to 11.1 mmol/L greater than the target levels, it may suggest that what you just drank is causing you to urinate more and absorb less sugar in your kidneys.

Hypoglycemia cannot be determined with urine glucose testing since a negative urine glucose outcome may occur when the glucose level is 0 to 180 mg/dL or higher. You might think you are in great shape just because test results are always negative. The reality is that, for elderly and renal disease diabetics, kidney thresholds are relatively high and produce false negative results in the presence of an unsafely high glucose level.

KETONE TESTING

When ketones are found in the urine, it means that the patient's Type 1 diabetes is worsening, and the possibility of DKA is very high. As insulin function deteriorates, there is a breakdown of stored fat to use for energy. Ketone bodies are the end result of this breakdown of fat, and they therefore end up in the blood and urine.

Patients usually use a urine dipstick, such as Ketostix or Chemstrip uK, to ascertain if they have ketonuria, or ketones in their urine. When ketones are present, the reagent pad on the strip turns a purplish color. One of the ketone bodies is acetone, which can be used interchangeably with the term *ketones.* Other strips are available on the market to measure the levels of glucose *and* ketones, including Keto-Diastix or Chemstrip uGK. If huge amounts of ketones are present, the color response on the strips may be difficult to recognize.

Patients with Type 1 diabetes, glucosuria (glucose in the urine), or chronic elevation of sugar levels above 240 mg/dL for two consecutive testing periods should check carefully for the presence of ketones in their urine. Ketone tests may be administered during pregnancy or in times of illness. Having a preexisting condition with diabetes or gestational diabetes also warrants ketone screenings.

GENERAL ASSESSMENT OF NEWLY DIAGNOSED DIABETICS

To understand a diagnosis of diabetes, we should identify the history, physical assessment, and underlying manifestations for a particular patient. These steps are customary in hospitals, clinics, and other health facilities. Hospitals need to know the degree of illness and the etiology, or the cause, of each of your medical conditions. Health care providers are usually concerned about prolonged hyperglycemia and other physical symptoms linked to diabetes.

Diabetics are typically asked to describe their symptoms, which may include the following:

- Polydipsia (excessive thirst)
- Polyuria (excessive urination)
- Polyphagia (excessive appetite)
- Dryness of the skin
- Blurred vision
- Weight loss
- Vaginal itching
- Wounds or ulcers that do not heal

Testing of blood glucose levels together with urine ketone levels may be necessary for those with Type 1 diabetes, who are noted for symptoms related to DKA, like ketonuria, Kussmaul respiration (labored breathing), orthostatic hypotension, and lethargy. Laboratory values are also checked for preexisting metabolic acidosis, which is indicated by low pH and bicarbonate levels and electrolyte imbalance.

If you have Type 2 diabetes, you will be assessed for possible signs of hyperglycemic hyperosmolar nonketotic syndrome (HHNS), like hypotension, altered sensory perception, seizures, and decreased turgor of the skin. Laboratory values are also monitored for hyperosmolality and electrolyte imbalance.

Visual deficits of the eye are also taken into consideration. Your doctor may do a rapid eye test by asking you to read the information on medication labels or insulin pens. You could be observed while eating and performing other activities, such as holding a syringe or a finger lancing instrument.

Neurological status can be evaluated through a patient's history of illnesses, speaking capacities, and ability to follow simple directional commands.

SHOULD EVERYONE GET TESTED FOR DIABETES?

The American Diabetes Association (ADA) recommends that people with various health conditions be tested for diabetes and prediabetes. The ADA also suggests that people forty-five and older be checked for diabetes, even if they don't report any risk factors like obesity or an ethnicity particularly prone to diabetes.

Here is a checklist that the ADA refers to when determining whether someone is at risk for developing diabetes:

- Physical inactivity
- A family history of diabetes
- The following ethnic origins: African, Alaska Native, American Indian, Asian, Hispanic/Latino, or Pacific Islander
- Current or previous hypertension readings of 140/90 mmHg and above
- Having an HDL, or "good" cholesterol, level under 35 mg/dL or a triglyceride level higher than 250 mg/dL
- Polycystic ovary syndrome (PCOS)
- Being told to have IFG or IGT during a previous examination
- Having a dark, velvety rash around the neck or armpits, also known as acanthosis nigricans
- A history of cardiovascular disease or other diseases involving the heart and blood vessels

Even when you are free of diabetes, it is advisable that you get checked for the above risk factors at least three times a year.

Patients with prediabetes must be tested again at least one to two years later to learn about the progress or deterioration of the condition. This can prevent Type 2 diabetes.

Correspondingly, when a woman is pregnant, her physician will test her during her first prenatal visit to determine if she has gestational diabetes and will order more tests if needed. Patients with gestational diabetes should be examined again six to twelve weeks after the baby's birth to find out if the disease has developed into Type 2 diabetes.

Children and teens are also prone to developing diabetes nowadays, so it is important to monitor the health of kids, especially if they are at risk. Testing for individuals aged ten and older should be done at least every two years. Keep in mind that testing your health on a regular schedule is part of a holistic approach to treating your health.

WHAT HAPPENS AFTER DIAGNOSIS OF PREDIABETES OR DIABETES?

Once diagnosed with prediabetes or diabetes, a patient may experience mental alterations and mixed feelings. No matter what your feelings and thoughts are, it is strongly advised that you take your mind off the worries that come with diabetes. Have confidence in your diagnosis and treatment program in spite of the lack of a permanent cure for diabetes. As you learn about the condition itself, there is a good chance that you will also learn how to handle the manifestations that occur with it.

At the moment, no one can make diabetes vanish into thin air, but you do have the power to prevent complications. Soon you will understand how great the power of the mind is in fighting this debilitating disease. Know that the earlier you have your diabetes diagnosed, the better your chances are of resisting it.

Patients usually have their diabetes treated initially by a general practitioner, internist, or family physician. Depending on the severity of the situation, you may be better off having your diabetes treated by an endocrinologist.

An endocrinologist is a physician who specializes in internal medicine and then endocrinology, the medical specialty concerning hormone health. Some endocrinologists deal with nondiabetic hormones like the thyroid and adrenal glands, while others specialize in diabetes and insulin.

Endocrinologists are usually located in urban areas, where larger institutions are available to cater to advanced endocrine situations. If you live in a rural area and would like to seek the service of an endocrinologist, don't worry. There are plenty of diabetes educators in far-away regions that can refer you to a nearby doctor to help you with your condition.

INSULIN RESISTANCE TESTING

Since diabetes is related to the malfunctioning of insulin, testing for insulin resistance is of paramount importance. Let's consider some of the factors leading a person to insulin resistance:

- Being overweight, with a BMI of more than twenty-five
- Very low HDL (good) cholesterol—less than 40 mg/dL for males and less than 50 mg/dL for females
- A very high triglyceride level—more than 150 mg/dL
- A high blood pressure reading—more than 130/80 mmHg
- A greater than normal fasting blood glucose level—above 100 mg/dL
- Protein in the urine

In addition to the factors mentioned above, the diagnostic tests described in this chapter tell more about the likelihood of diabetes in an individual. To be able to understand diabetes tests, we have to consider things across the board. Most screenings are just tools to aid us in determining the severity of certain factors, but it is nonetheless very important to have a deeper knowledge of these tests.

DIAGNOSING HYPOGLYCEMIA

In diagnosing hypoglycemia, you must first rule out other causes, like an insulinoma, which is a tumor in the pancreas. Insulinomas cause the production of a very high amount of insulin. They may also lead to other diseases, such as peritoneal tumors, adrenal insufficiency, kidney failure, or congestive heart failure.

We talked earlier about SMBG. The best way to know if a person has hypoglycemia is through self-testing at home. You can begin by testing yourself early in the morning. Remember to take the test first thing in the morning after you wake up.

DIAGNOSING POLYCYSTIC OVARIAN SYNDROME

Diabetic women can fall victim to a condition known as polycystic ovarian syndrome (PCOS). Risk factors for this disease include, but are not limited to, central obesity, a family history of diabetes, irregular periods, hair growth resembling that of males, and fertility treatment. Yes, the treatment of one problem can be a risk factor for another.

PCOS can be frustrating for any female patient because it is often left undiagnosed, leading to infertility and other stresses in those inflicted. This disease can also result from the insulin resistance of being a diabetic. However, not all causes of PCOS have to do with insulin resistance, and as of today medical researchers have not been able to come up with a 100 percent foolproof screening procedure for PCOS.

Insulin resistance is associated with PCOS, so go ahead and test yourself for insulin resistance if you suspect it based on your symptoms. Remember that symptoms like irregular menstruation, acne, excessive facial hair, and the like will also be treated once the insulin resistance has been isolated.

To confirm PCOS beyond the diagnostic tools we have mentioned, physicians usually make use of blood work. This begins with a fasting sugar level test and a fasting lipid panel. The metabolic syndrome, kidneys, and liver function are also diagnosed. In some cases, the liver function turns out to be uncharacteristic in the presence of insulin resistance.

A pregnancy test is also performed. If the woman is pregnant, she might have difficulties with childbirth. Endocrine organs, such as the adrenal, thyroid, and pituitary glands, get evaluated to make sure that the symptoms being experienced aren't really accounted for by other sicknesses.

Prolactin, a hormone responsible for lactation, is used to check brain and pituitary gland function. Thyroid function tests are also taken into account.

Free and total testosterone, a male hormone substance, is closely monitored along with DHEAS levels. DHEAS (dehydroepiandrosterone sulfate) is a medical screening used for diagnosing polycystic ovarian syndrome. If hormones are found to be out of sync in the DHEAS, there will be further examination and treatment. Doctors may still choose to do an ultrasound of the ovaries, but this is not absolutely necessary to confirm PCOS.

CALCULATING THE BODY MASS INDEX (BMI)

Since being overweight leads to a greater risk of acquiring insulin resistance, prediabetes, and diabetes, learning how to calculate the body mass index (BMI) is very useful. There are easier ways to determine body weight, such as the use of commercially available scales, but we can be more attuned to diabetes by using the specific values that the medical world uses to compare height and weight.

Basic guidelines indicate that if you weigh 175 pounds, for example, your height to match that should be around six feet tall. On the other hand, when an individual with the same weight is shorter, the situation is much different. This is why we need to dig a little further into BMI.

To properly compute BMI, divide your weight in kilograms by your height in meters squared (kg/m^2). It is much easier to calculate BMI through plug-and-play websites, unless you prefer manual computation.

Generally, a BMI less than 25 is deemed satisfactory, but a person who has a very low BMI, like 17, is occasionally diagnosed as underweight. The thin models we see on television have BMIs of around seventeen or eighteen. Once your BMI reaches more than 25, you are considered overweight; if it surpasses 30, you could be suffering from obesity.

The Links between Apples and Pears

Most diabetics who are overweight tend to have an *O* or apple shape. This is of course a metaphorical expression, but it does serve as a strong reminder of what can happen to the physique of a person when he or she becomes obese. Overweight people differ in body shape depending on factors unrelated to obesity itself. In some diabetics, fats are concentrated in the middle of the body. This is known as central obesity or apple-shaped obesity. In this type of obesity, the person has relatively slim upper and lower extremities.

Meanwhile, other diabetics have fat all over, with more fat concentrated in the buttocks, hips, and thighs. Their obesity is referred to as pear-shaped or *A*-shaped obesity.

Insulin resistant patients and diabetes victims generally suffer from the apple-shaped form of obesity. These people have a higher risk of heart disease and diabetes, whereas patients with a pear shape are at minor risk. There is a bulky placement of fat on the liver, pancreas, and intestines in people suffering from central obesity. The inner fat can cause various complications with internal organs, triggering insulin resistance (Type 2 diabetes) and other forms of diabetes.

CHOLESTEROL AND TRIGLYCERIDE LEVELS

Aside from blood glucose levels, insulin resistance is a crucial factor that contributes to cholesterol levels and the incidence of heart attacks. How can you have a heart attack after a doctor has told you that your cholesterol is at a healthy level? First, there are two types of cholesterol found in our bodies, referred to as low-density lipoprotein (LDL) and high-density lipoprotein

(HDL). Low-density protein is commonly labeled *bad* cholesterol, while high-density lipoprotein is the good cholesterol.

In combination with other abnormalities of our circulatory vessels, inflammation and coagulation caused by insulin resistance can lead to a higher risk of having a heart attack. Elevated LDL levels pose a great risk to diabetics, because LDL leads to the occlusion of arteries.

Heart attacks are generally caused by the collection of cholesterol along the inner walls of our blood vessels. *Plaque* is the name for hazardous cholesterol deposits. Plaque is associated with abnormal fat and cholesterol levels in the vascular system, and the best way to measure its existence is by doing a fasting lipid panel.

Four major figures are recorded when measuring your cholesterol, the first of which is total cholesterol. This value is usually below 200 mg/dL. A higher level of cholesterol is linked to insulin resistance, especially when sugar is in excess of 150 mg/dL. You also have to watch out for triglyceride levels, which bring on hypertriglyceremia when too high. You could gain a serious amount of weight as a result. Sugar levels are equally affected, since glucose plays a large role in fat metabolism.

An unusual upswing of lipids in the body is the main reason that cardiac disease sometimes precedes diabetes. When triglyceride levels are elevated, the good (HDL) cholesterol levels decrease, and the bad (LDL) cholesterol turns smaller and denser. These triglyceride levels do not necessarily mean danger at first, but they may result in serious clinical consequences in the end.

Lipid panel instruments can separate the data on good and bad cholesterol. The LDL level must be held below 100 mg/dL, but studies have shown that 70 mg/dL is a more desirable level. Good cholesterol should be more than 40 mg/dL. When the level goes below 40 mg/dL for males and 50 mg/dL for females, it increases the risk of insulin resistance and cardiac disease. When you have a lot of HDL cholesterol moving around inside you, bad cholesterol is taken away from the arteries and is led to the liver.

BLOOD PRESSURE IN DIABETICS

Countless diabetics suffer from clinical complications that include abnormalities in blood pressure. As the key player in your own health who can learn and develop good health habits, you have to equip yourself with the necessary "weapons" to counteract these symptoms.

High blood pressure, or hypertension, is very common in people with prediabetes, but ironically, there are currently no direct statistical relationships between hypertension and high risk for prediabetes. If you were to evaluate any number of patients with prediabetes at any given time, you would notice that many have issues with blood pressure, but some do not. Moreover, even when a person has low blood pressure, it does not mean that person does not have prediabetes.

Various hormones are available for regulating blood pressure. Diabetics with insulin resistance usually experience high blood pressure (above 130/80 mmHg). When there is high blood pressure or hypertension involved, there are added stressors affecting the walls of the heart and blood vessels, in addition to the brain and kidneys.

Let's consider the monitoring procedures on a broader scale. When measuring blood pressure, you should sit calmly on a chair with your legs uncrossed. Place your testing arm at the level of your heart. Make sure the blood pressure cuff fits your arm comfortably.

Blood pressure cuffs come in different sizes—child, adult, and thigh—but the standard size usually works for anyone who isn't overweight. Meanwhile, a thigh cuff might be required for obese diabetics. A child's cuff may work well for smaller patients.

Misplacing the cuff on the arm or using incorrect sizes elicits inaccurate blood pressure readings. Familiarize yourself on how to record blood pressure, whether your own or that of another diabetic.

Remember that there are two different figures involved with blood pressure. Blood pressure readings are always written thus: 130/80, or 130 over 80. The top number represents your systolic blood pressure, which signals a contraction of the heart's ventricles. Systolic blood pressure refers to when there is a much higher contractive force in the heart. During systole, the heart is pumping out blood to be distributed by the vascular system to other areas of the body. The systolic number should always be higher than the one below it. The number below the systolic pressure is the diastolic pressure. It refers to the fluid pressure present when the heart muscle is between beats.

DIAGNOSTIC MEASURES IN ACUTE COMPLICATIONS OF DIABETES

There are various diagnostic procedures involved when speaking of acute, or sudden, complications associated with diabetes. We'll go through them in a little more detail in upcoming chapters.

Hypoglycemia

Hypoglycemia is considered an acute complication in which your blood glucose levels are less than 100mg/dL. Hypoglycemic manifestations may occur in all types of diabetes, but the way the body reacts to these fluctuations varies from person to person. If you are used to having sugar levels of around 220 mg/dL but currently have 120 mg/dL, you may experience various symptoms related to hypoglycemia. This is one reason that routine monitoring of sugar levels is highly advised.

Diabetic Ketoacidosis (DKA)

When affected by DKA, blood glucose levels may be as low as 300 mg/dL and as high as 800 mg/dL (16.6 to 44.4 mmol/L). Depending on how hydrated you are, you could experience very low glucose levels with diabetic ketoacidosis, while others might have very high values of 1,000 mg/dL (55.5 mmol/L) or more. The extent of your DKA symptoms does not always depend on sugar levels. Diabetics may experience severe acidosis but have only a moderately high glucose level, while some may have no manifestations of DKA but glucose levels of 400 to 500 mg/dL (22.2 to 27.7 mmol/L).

Ketoacidosis can be discovered through low serum bicarbonate (0 to 15 mEq/L) and a low pH range of 6.8 to 7.3. A low PCO_2 range, like 10 to 30 mmHg, signals a possibility of Kussmaul respirations. Kussmaul respirations involve deep breathing at a desirable or heightened rate when a diabetic is experiencing metabolic acidosis.

Sodium and potassium values are likewise very low, normal, or high, depending on your level of hydration. Plasma concentrations of these electrolytes may have been decreased and may need to be increased as soon as possible.

Creatinine, a waste product of metabolism, is excessive in DKA patients who do not have any problems staying hydrated. Levels of blood urea nitrogen (BUN), hemoglobin, and hematocrit constitute a major concern in such individuals. When the individual is rehydrated, there will continue to be elevated levels of the serum creatinine and BUN, especially in those with renal insufficiency.

Diagnosis of Hyperglycemic Hyperosmolar Nonketotic Syndrome

To diagnose hyperglycemic hyperosmolar nonketotic syndrome (HHNS), detailed laboratory analyses are performed. These procedures include measures of blood glucose, electrolytes, BUN, and serum osmolality, as well as a complete blood count and arterial blood gas (ABG) analysis. Total sugar levels may be as high as 600 to 1,200 mg/dL, and the fluid osmolarity could reach levels in excess of 350 mOsm/kg. Electrolyte and BUN levels are almost the same as for diabetics suffering from severe dehydration. Mental status shifts and focal neurologic irregularities may slowly begin to surface. There may be severe hallucinations, indicating cerebral dehydration as a by-product of hyperosmolarity.

DIAGNOSTIC MEASURES IN CHRONIC
COMPLICATIONS OF DIABETES

To be successful in the fight against diabetes, you must understand the pathways of short-term and long-term forms of the disease. Knowledge of the following diagnostics is required to position yourself effectively against diabetes.

Microvascular Complications

To diagnose microvascular complications and diabetic retinopathy, the doctor will physically examine your eye using an ophthalmoscope, or by a specific technique known as fluorescein angiography. These procedures reveal the progression of different types of retinopathy. Fluorescein angiography lets you know the severity of any retinopathy you may have. A dye is injected into the arm vein and is distributed to different areas via circulation, mainly to the vessels located in the retina of the eye. Through this technique, the ophthalmologist, or eye doctor, employs special instruments to see the retinal vessels in vivid detail, providing vital information that would otherwise be impossible to extract using just an ophthalmoscope.

Side effects of this dye procedure include the following:

- Experiencing nausea while the dye is being injected
- Discoloration of the skin
- Occasional allergic reactions, usually in the form of hives or itching
- Fluorescent or yellow urine, lasting anywhere from twelve to twenty-four hours

Nephropathy as a Chronic Complication

To detect nephropathy, it is important to determine the presence of a distinct protein seeping into the urine called albumin. With the tendency of diabetics to go undiagnosed for years, a diabetic may have nephropathy without even knowing it. When you have microalbuminuria, the chance of developing clinical nephropathy increases by more than 85 percent. If microalbuminuria does not emerge, your chances are less than 5 percent.

Early detection of microalbuminuria is accomplished by analyzing a twelve- to twenty-four-hour urine sample. As a diabetic, you should have your urine checked for microalbuminuria every year. Once the microalbumin level exceeds 30 mg per twenty-four hours during two consecutive examinations, a corresponding treatment will be administered. Serum creatinine and

BUN levels are examined when a urine dipstick reveals a consistently positive albumin test.

For diabetics with renal disease, testing for the presence of cardiac symptoms and other complications is strongly recommended. Testing in this regard entails the injection of special dyes that stain positive for microalbumin. Since hypertension is likely to occur in both diabetics and nondiabetics who are in the early stages of renal disease, constant monitoring of blood pressure is recommended. Around 50 percent of people with diabetes will experience hypertension for unknown reasons. Thus it is safe to assume that if you have diabetes and hypertension, you may also be in the initial stages of kidney disease. However, you should always get the right diagnostic and screening procedures encouraged by your doctor before reaching any such medical conclusions.

• 5 •

Treatment Options

$\mathcal{S}$haring the information about treating diabetes is a good way of making people more aware of the disease. There are five main components in the therapeutic treatment of diabetes: nutritional management, exercise, monitoring, pharmacological therapy, and education.

The goal of therapeutic measures is to achieve conventional glucose levels (euglycemia), to lower the incidence of vascular and neuropathic complications, to reduce hypoglycemia, and to affect the patient's lifestyle and activities as little as possible. Certainly, the American Diabetes Association strongly advises those with diabetes on the importance of controlling their blood sugar.

To determine the importance of blood glucose control, the Diabetes Control and Complications Trial (DCCT) performed a ten-year prospective clinical trial beginning in 1983. Through this trial, the effect of strict glucose control on the development of retinopathy, nephropathy, and neuropathy was investigated. More than 1,400 patients with Type 1 diabetes were randomly assigned specific treatments, including (1) one to two insulin injections a day, or three to four for intensive treatment, and (2) insulin pump therapy, with ample monitoring of blood glucose.

According to the results of this study, strict sugar regulation at standard or near-normal level cuts down the chances of getting retinopathy and neuropathy. It also holds back early symptoms of nephropathy, microalbuminuria, and albuminuria.

With this intensive therapy, however, comes a higher risk of acquiring severe hypoglycemia, falling into a coma, or having a seizure episode. As an upshot, there must be careful monitoring during the intensive therapy period, along with education of the patient and family, to prepare them for taking favorable health measures when the time comes.

BEGINNING TREATMENT

After being diagnosed with diabetes, you may come to feel like monitoring your illness is a full-time job. Acquiring all this new information may make you feel like you are back in school. You may feel overwhelmed with scheduling doctor's appointments, dieting the right way, monitoring your blood glucose levels daily, and other routines associated with the condition. But all of this is really to ensure your good health. It is true that diabetes always causes trouble in your life, but through discipline and proper motivation, you get used to all of the strange routines you have to slip into your life.

FINDING GOOD HEALTH CARE CAN BE AS REALISTIC AS TEEN FICTION

Since diabetes is a complex disease that can develop into other illnesses, and vice versa, if you educate yourself on the best treatment methods, there is a greater chance that you can control your condition.

Besides educating yourself on the disease and monitoring your blood glucose levels, you should also get to know the person taking care of you. Remember, you don't have to be the only participant in your treatment. You can decide whether or not you are satisfied with the treatment you are receiving from physicians or other health care providers. Remember that your own wellness is at stake, so you should be knowledgeable of the options available and use them to your advantage.

BUILDING THE DIABETES DREAM TEAM

When you suspect diabetes, the first person to seek out is a regular doctor, who will be in charge of your diagnosis, evaluation, and treatment. Once you start seeing your doctor, make sure their knowledge and treatment techniques are to your liking. Your primary care physician should be compassionate and forthcoming about your condition.

A routine medical visit generally takes seven to twelve minutes. The visit will usually include the following:

- Blood pressure measurement
- Weight check
- A brief interview

- Prescription for medication
- Nonpharmaceutical therapy referrals, if needed
- Scheduling of the next appointment

Because of all the things that need to be done during a routine visit, your overall treatment may require more than one physician. A diabetic may need multiple health care providers to help boost wellness, control symptoms, and provide you with services that require various treatments.

Who comprises your health care team aside from your primary care doctor? Well, you could be referred to an endocrinologist when push comes to shove. You may also need a diabetes educator, perhaps a nurse or a nutritionist, or maybe a certified diabetes educator who specializes in teaching patients how to manage the disease.

As you experience specific symptoms, like eye problems, you might be referred to an ophthalmologist, or eye doctor, who knows how to deal with diabetic eye diseases, such as diabetic retinopathy. Meanwhile, a podiatrist (foot doctor) might be called in to help you if you suffer from neuropathy, numbness, or severe foot pain.

MANAGING NUTRITION

The foundational success of diabetes management lies primarily with diet, weight control, and nutrition. The goal is to control the total caloric intake and hold body weight within a reasonable range based on BMI.

Reversing hyperglycemia and reaching weight goals is essential in dealing with Type 2 diabetes, but sometimes this is no easy task. Managing diabetes through nutrition involves various approaches. Therefore a registered dietitian who specializes in diabetes management should be consulted. Other health care workers, like nurses, should also have knowledge of the dietary requirements of diabetics if a dietitian is not around.

According to the ADA, nutritional goals for the diabetic should include the following:

- Information on the foods needed for optimal nutrition
- A diet that meets the individual's energy needs
- Achieving and supporting a reasonable weight
- Avoiding wide daily fluctuations in blood glucose levels and keeping them at near-normal levels
- Keeping serum lipid levels low to reduce the risk of macrovascular disease

Sticking to proper amounts of calories and carbohydrates during meals is important if you are a diabetic required to take insulin for controlling sugar levels. Consistent intervals between meal times, and snacks if needed, will keep away hypoglycemic reactions and can help regain control of glucose levels.

For Type 2 diabetics who are obese, losing weight is just as important as preventing the disease from occurring. As previously stated, an overweight individual has a BMI above 25, while a medically obese person has a BMI of 30 or higher. For obese patients who do not take insulin, monitoring meal contents and following consistent meal schedules is not as critical. Reducing the caloric content is, however, extremely important. This does not mean that meals should be skipped in an effort to deplete calories, however, because when you forgo a meal, you are actually increasing the workload of your pancreas.

Adhering to such a strict meal plan for a long period can be very challenging. Obese diabetics tend to adhere to the plan more easily if the restriction of calories is done at a moderate pace, rather than stressing the person's limitations right at the very beginning. In dealing with obesity, it is crucial that group support and behavioral therapy be combined with the incorporation of new dietary habits, education, and continuous nutritional counseling.

TREATING DIABETES WITH SPECIAL MEAL PLANS

The meal plan is an important part of managing diabetes. A successful meal plan must take into consideration food preferences, lifestyle, frequency of meals, and even ethnic or cultural background. For those who are taking intensive insulin therapy, the timing and content of the meals can be adjusted to allow for changes in eating and exercise routines. Patients taking more advanced insulin therapy, such as insulin analogs, insulin algorithms, or insulin pumps, can exercise greater flexibility in their schedules.

Your eating habits are also important to consider when constructing a diabetic meal plan. The clinical dietitian will make use of different tools, approaches, and materials that incorporate the specific diabetic's eating habits. He or she may educate you on adhering to their meal plan when eating in restaurants, checking food labels, exercising, coping with ailments, or other situations.

Caloric Requirements

To determine the proper caloric intake, the energy needs and the caloric requirements of the patient are first computed on the basis of age, gender, height, and weight. Physical activity is factored in to provide a reasonable number of calories needed to maintain your desired weight. If you wish to lose one to two pounds a week, you need to subtract approximately five hundred to one thousand calories from your daily diet. The remaining caloric intake is divided up into carbohydrates, proteins, and fats. Furthermore, the information above can get you halfway to devising a standardized meal plan for yourself.

Your health care provider may provide you with the *Exchange Lists for Meal Planning*, an information packet showing the proper distribution of calories needed to boast a successful diet. The packet provides a lot of helpful information, considering the fact that every meal and snack needs to be monitored and measured carefully. This is why the meal plan should be structured around the diabetic's individual lifestyle.

For younger people with Type 1 diabetes, the goal is to have an adequate supply of calories that can support their continued growth and development. Because some younger people may be underweight due to severe hypoglycemia, they could have a high-calorie diet to make up for the weight loss.

From a more detailed perspective, a diabetic diet focuses on providing the following necessary nutrients: carbohydrates, proteins, and fats. Carbohydrates have the biggest effect on blood glucose levels since they are easily digested and rapidly converted into glucose. This is different from most other nutrients. In the past, professional health care personnel believed that diabetic diets should contain more proteins and fats to decrease postprandial levels of carbohydrates. Regrettably, this practice merely leads to complications that sometimes include cardiovascular disease.

WORKING OUT AS A DIABETIC

One of the most important aspects of diabetic treatment is exercise, which when done in the right manner can help maintain good levels of blood sugars and reduce the risk of cardiovascular disease.

Exercise can significantly increase the sugar uptake of the muscles and improve the utilization of insulin. This can lead to better circulation and muscle tone. Exercises like resistance or strength training, including weight lifting, can enhance lean muscle mass while simultaneously increasing the resting metabolic weight.

Exercise promotes a reduction of weight, which is crucial for indirectly controlling diabetes. It helps relieve stress and enhances a person's general well-being. It also raises high-density lipoprotein levels and controls total cholesterol and triglyceride amounts in the cardiovascular system.

Considerations and Precautions

This may surprise you, but exercise undoubtedly has its drawbacks and precautions. Diabetics with sugar levels exceeding 250 mg/dL (14 mmol/L) and who have ketones in their urine must not work out too vigorously unless their urine tests are negative for the presence of ketones and their sugar levels are sound. When warnings are ignored, exercising generally will boost the secretion of glucose, paving the way for a much higher sugar level than wanted.

If you take insulin and plan on working out, remember to eat a fifteen-gram carb snack, fruit, or even food with complex carbohydrates and proteins once in a while. This should be done ahead of any moderate exercise so you can avoid an unexpected bout of hypoglycemia.

The amount of food needed before exercising depends almost entirely on the level of sugars present. In some cases, there is no need for a preexercise snack if you routinely perform the exercise one to two hours after a meal. On the other hand, some individuals need to have the extra calories on backup regardless of the length of the exercise. If additional food is required for exercising, it does not have to be deducted from the regular meal plan.

Diabetes patients who are on insulin therapy should also know that hypoglycemia can occur several hours after exercise. To prevent postexercise hypoglycemia after a strenuous or prolonged workout, the diabetic may need to have a snack at the end of the session. Diabetics who exercise may also need a snack before bedtime.

Occasionally a patient may need to limit the dosage of insulin when they exercise. Once the effective levels of insulin are determined, you have to be able to regulate your own insulin dosages when needed. If this is impossible, you can stick with specific instructions on exercising.

Patients with Type 2 diabetes should combine exercise with dietary measures that will improve glucose metabolism and enhance the loss of unwanted fat. This will improve insulin absorption and may even prevent the need for insulin or oral antidiabetic agents. There may be a return to glucose tolerance. Patients with Type 2 diabetes who are not prescribed direct insulin or an oral agent may not need the extra food before exercising.

RECOMMENDATIONS WHEN EXERCISING

It is recommended that diabetes patients exercise at the same time every day and for the same amount of time. Sporadic exercise sessions are not recommended. However, those suffering from complications such as autonomic neuropathy, retinopathy, sensorimotor neuropathy, and cardiovascular disease may have to alter their exercise routines since regular exercise can trigger complications such as diabetic retinopathy, which in turn may increase the risk of hemorrhage in the eye. Those with ischemic heart disease may be at risk for developing angina or myocardial infarction and not be aware of it. Last but not least, avoid trauma to the lower extremities, particularly if you are experiencing numbness associated with neuropathy.

A slow and gradual increase in exercise is advised. Walking is a safe bet because it is a highly effective exercise that requires few or no special devices and can be done anywhere, at any time.

Consult your doctor before beginning any exercise routine. Health care providers from time to time may alert you to precautions and restrictions you should be mindful of before taking on an exercise regimen. It is also recommended that patients with at least two risk factors for diabetes, or those over thirty years of age, undergo an exercise stress test to rule out hypertension and high cholesterol. Doctors may make note of any obesity, smoking, or family history of cardiovascular disease before permitting someone to exercise. The same applies to the typical diabetic with a sedentary lifestyle or an abnormal resting EKG.

PHARMACOLOGICAL THERAPY: WHEN NATURE CALLS FOR DRUGS

As you may know, insulin is a hormone secreted by beta cells in the islets of Langerhans. It serves to decrease the levels of blood glucose through its utilization in fat, muscle, and liver cells. Without a sufficient amount of insulin in the body, however, other diabetes medications are vital.

Insulin Therapy and Preparations

In Type 1 diabetes, there is a general loss of the ability to produce insulin, so other sources of insulin must be administered for the rest of the patient's life. In Type 2 diabetes, insulin may be prescribed as needed for a long period of time if oral medications and changes in diet prove insufficient. Insulin may also be prescribed during periods of illness, infection, surgery, pregnancy, or other stressful situations.

Some diabetics do well by special diet alone or by a diet paired with medication. In other cases, insulin injections are required two or more times a day to regulate sugar levels. Thus, to determine the necessary insulin dosage, frequent self-monitoring of circulatory glucose must be performed. There are also various types of insulin available on the market, but they all do relatively the same job. Insulin samples only differ in their chemical properties. These properties include time for absorption, course of action, and source of origin.

Based on the above characteristics, insulin is grouped into various categories. Human insulin preparations, for instance, have a shorter duration compared to insulin derived from animals. Rapid-acting preparations, like insulin lispro (Humalog) and semi insulin (Novolog), possess sugar-fighting components that produce quicker effects. These drugs, however, stay in the bloodstream for a shorter amount of time than regular insulin. They have an onset of five to fifteen minutes, with peak action at one hour following the injection, and they stay active for about two hours. Diabetics using rapid-acting insulin should eat no more than five to fifteen minutes after an insulin injection.

Patients with Type 1, gestational, and some forms of Type 2 diabetes should also take long-acting insulin to keep the total sugar amounts at target levels. Basal insulin is also necessary for keeping the levels consistent despite irregular meal habits. Intermediate-acting insulin serves a similar purpose to basal insulin, but it is normally separated into two injections given every twelve hours.

Short-acting insulin, designated with an *R* on the bottle, is now available and has an onset time of thirty minutes to an hour. It also has a peak of two to three hours and an action time of four to six hours. Regular insulin, also denoted by *R*, is a clear solution and is often given twenty to thirty minutes prior to meals. It can be administered alone or together with long-acting insulin. Examples of regular insulin include Novolin R, Humulin R, and Iletin Regular.

Intermediate-acting insulins, also known as neutral protamine Hagedorn (NPH) insulin or lente insulin, have an onset time of three to four hours, a peak of four to twelve hours, and an active duration of sixteen to twenty hours. This type of cloudy-looking insulin has a course of action similar to that of long-acting insulin. If NPH or lente insulin is taken alone, it is not necessary to wait thirty minutes before eating. However, it is vital that during the peak and onset the individual eat some type of food. Some examples of NPH insulins are Humulin N, Iletin NPH, and Novolin N. Novolin L, Iletin L, and Humulin L are types of lente insulin.

Ultralente insulins, or long-acting insulins, are called peakless insulins because they have slow, prolonged, and sustained effects, as opposed to sharp and definite peaks of action. The onset of this form of insulin is six to eight hours, with a peak of twelve to sixteen hours, and a duration of twenty to thirty hours.

Peakless basal insulin includes insulin glargine (Lantus). It is metabolized slowly over a twenty-four-hour period and can be administered once per day, usually at bedtime. Since this type of insulin is really in an acidic suspension with a pH of 4, it cannot be combined with other insulins. If combined, precipitation will occur and cause pain. Lente/ultralente insulin is no longer used in the United States.

Inhaled insulin may soon be approved for use in the near future. This insulin is administered in the form of a very fine powder inhaled from a device similar to an asthma inhaler. It is breathed in prior to meals.

Sources of insulin   In the past, insulin samples were acquired from the pancreas of cows and pigs. "Human insulin," manufactured via recombinant DNA technology, is the most common form of insulin in use today.

Insulin manufacturers   In the United States, two companies are the primary manufacturers of insulin: Eli Lilly and Novo Nordisk. The insulins produced by these companies are interchangeable because the concentration (e.g., U-100) and type (e.g., NPH) are very similar. These insulins may be sold under various brand names, so the human insulin that is used might be either Humulin N or Novolin N.

Considerations when Administering Insulin

Holistic treatment protocols involving insulin usually require one to four injections a day and may combine short-acting insulin with long-acting insulin depending on how the pancreas is currently functioning. Operating at its peak, the pancreas secretes insulin throughout the day and night. After food is digested and blood sugars subsequently rise, insulin is secreted in large amounts to compensate for the elevated glucose that resulted when food was taken in. Once-a-day insulin injections are the simplest way to deal with the food intake and various patterns of activity.

Before varying their insulin dosage, patients should know how to interpret their SMBG numbers and record their carbohydrates. When you do this, you are also able to change the timing and content of your food intake in relation to your exercise routines. However, the process requires quite a bit of commitment and discipline. The individual must have sufficient education and training and be monitored by his or her doctor to keep optimal glucose levels.

Insulin on a Larger Scale

There are two general approaches to insulin therapy: conventional and intensive. The conventional approach may be used to avoid the possible acute complications of diabetes, like hypoglycemia and symptomatic hyperglycemia. A combination of intermediate- and short-acting insulin may be used for daily injections. Those who use the conventional approach often have deviant glucose levels but don't vary their meal patterns or activity levels.

The conventional approach is recommended for diabetics who are any of the following:

- Terminally ill
- Weak
- Elderly
- Unwilling to monitor their glucose
- Physically unable to monitor their glucose
- Opposed to nontraditional methods

The second approach is much more intensive. It involves a more complicated insulin regimen to control glucose levels. Under this approach, there is a greater chance of preventing long-term complications, and the individual has more flexibility in shifting the daily dosage. This depends on eating patterns, illness, and stress, all of which can affect your sugar values.

Not all diabetics need rigid blood glucose monitoring, but for those undergoing intensive treatment, such an approach may help ease the risk of severe hypoglycemia.

Complications of Insulin Therapy

Approximately one to two hours after insulin administration, diabetics may experience a local allergic reaction in the form of redness, swelling, and tenderness at the site of the injection. These reactions usually occur at the beginning phases of therapy and will disappear with continued insulin use. Allergic reactions related to insulin therapy are less common today due to the use of human insulin instead of animal insulin. Nonetheless, when allergic reactions do occur, the physician usually prescribes taking an antihistamine an hour before the injection.

Systemic allergic reactions are rare, but if they do occur, it will appear as a local skin reaction that gradually turns into generalized urticaria, or hives. Treatment for this condition involves desensitization, whereby insulin doses are administered in trivial amounts at first that are later elevated.

Lipodystrophy is a change in the size or shape of the area around the injection, usually near fatty tissue. It may appear as a slight dimpling or a deeper pitting of the subcutaneous fat. Again, due to the use of human insulin today, this reaction has almost been eliminated.

Lipohypertrophy is the development of fibrous and fatty masses at the injection site. It is the result of using the same injection site over and over again. If the site gets scarred, absorption of insulin may be delayed. It is always a good idea to change injection sites occasionally. If you experience such symptoms, you should wait for the hypertrophy to disappear before reapplying the insulin.

Insulin Resistance

Owing to the fact that insulin resistance is directly related to so many other diseases, you should know about therapy techniques that help to prevent it. Insulin resistance is usually brought on by obesity, and the most commonly recommended prevention method is unquestionably weight loss. In clinical insulin resistance, there must be two hundred units or more of insulin daily. People who take insulin sometimes develop immune antibodies that bind to the insulin and deplete the levels that are ready to be used. All types of animal insulin, and even some human insulin (but to a lesser degree), result in the production of insulin antibodies.

Very few insulin resistant diabetics turn out to have high levels of these antibodies. For treatment, more concentrated insulin preparations, such as U-500, are needed. To prevent the body from manufacturing antibodies, prednisone is usually prescribed, frequently followed by a gradual reduction of insulin over time.

ALTERNATIVES IN DELIVERING INSULIN

Insulin Pens

Insulin pens have prefilled cartridges of 150 to 300 units of insulin that are loaded into a pen-shaped tool. A disposable needle is then attached to the device to inject the insulin. The user dials the appropriate dose or pushes a button that increases the amount of insulin administered in single or double increments. The advantage of using this type of injection is that you don't need to have insulin bottles or draw up insulin prior to every injection. This is recommended for people who have to inject only one type of insulin at a time, such as a pre-meal regular insulin dose taken three times a day followed by neutral protamine Hagedorn (NPH) insulin at bedtime.

Pens are convenient for patients using premixed insulin and for diabetics who are constantly on the go. They are also recommended for diabetics with impaired manual dexterity or with visual or cognitive difficulties. Traditional syringes can be difficult for these patients to use.

Jet Injectors

Jet injections administer insulin in a very fine stream through the skin using high pressure. These devices, however, are more expensive than those mentioned previously because they require special training to use. It should also be noted that jet injectors may alter the rate of absorption and the peak insulin activity, and may render the insulin ineffective to a certain extent. Overall, the absorption rate is faster with this method, but a number of patients experience bruising.

Insulin Pumps

Insulin pumps are small, externally worn devices that perform similar functions to the pancreas. These pumps have a three-milliliter syringe connected to a long, narrow lumen tube with a needle or Teflon catheter attached at the end. The needle or catheter is then inserted into the subcutaneous tissue, most commonly around the abdomen. It is secured with tape or transparent dressing. The pump is worn on a belt or in a pocket. For some women, the device is tucked into the front or side of a bra or into a garter belt wrapped around the thigh. The needle or catheter must be changed approximately every three days.

Fast-acting lispro insulin is administered with an insulin pump. It is given at the basal rate immediately before or after meals. Depending on the needs of the diabetic, the continuous basal rate is usually about one-half to two units per hour. When the individual activates the pump by pushing a series of buttons, a dose of insulin is administered. The patient selects the amount of insulin depending on his or her current sugar levels. The desired insulin quantity is also based on physical activity levels.

There are also many disadvantages to using insulin pumps. The flow of insulin can be interrupted if the tubing or needle becomes blocked, if the insulin supply is insufficient, or when the battery is depleted. This can lead to a higher risk of diabetic ketoacidosis (DKA).

With insulin pumps, there is also a greater probability of infection due to contamination of needle injection sites. Hypoglycemia is common with the insulin pump, and it is normally due to patient error instead of a problem with the pump itself. There is also a higher risk of developing hypoglycemia unawareness, which can result from a gradual decline of serum glucose levels, decreasing from 70 mg/dL (3.9 mmol/L) to 60 mg/dL (3.3 mmol/L).

Wearing such a device all day long is a huge inconvenience for many diabetics. You may be able to get away with disconnecting the device for a limited amount of time, based on individual needs and preference. When showering, exercising, or performing some other activity, you can and should remove the pump.

During pump therapy, the diabetic must be willing to monitor his or her blood glucose levels several times a day. Likewise, he or she must be psychologically stable and willing to live with such an indiscrete treatment option.

Today, most insurance companies cover the insulin pump's cost, but when coverage is not possible, it can be a significant financial burden on the diabetic. Luckily for those with Type 1 diabetes, Medicare actually covers most of the costs associated with insulin pumps.

Implantable and Inhalant Insulin Delivery

Due to advances in technology, studies have been conducted on the use of machines designed to deliver insulin through externally programmed insulin pumps that are implanted in the person's body. These devices monitor blood glucose levels and administer insulin automatically. Research is also being conducted on insulin that can be administered orally or in the form of sprays, inhalers, or skin patches.

Pancreatic Cell Transplants

The surge in diabetes throughout the world has also led to research on pancreas transplants. In fact, such operations have already been conducted, primarily for those receiving kidney transplants at the same time. The problem with this treatment, however, is potential transplant rejection and side effects of antirejection drugs and immunosuppressant therapy. A possible solution is the implantation of pancreatic islet cells capable of producing insulin. Proponents say this approach will make the procedure less extensive and will reduce the rate of immune system difficulties. Depending on how effective the resulting insulin is, a diabetic who has undergone transplant treatment may be able to enjoy a relatively unrestricted lifestyle.

ORAL ANTIDIABETIC MEDICATIONS

Oral agents can be effective for Type 2 diabetics whose condition is unmanageable through diet and exercise alone. An assortment of oral medications like sulfonylureas, biguanides, alpha glucosidase inhibitors, thiazolidinediones, and meglitinides have been developed in the United States. Several help the beta cells in the pancreas boost their production of insulin. These medications are discouraged in pregnant diabetics.

Sulfonylureas

Sulfonylureas force the pancreas to produce more insulin. They include the following drugs:

- Chlorpropamide (Diabinase)
- Tolazamide (Tolinase)
- Glipizide (Glucotrol)
- Tolbutamide (Orinase)
- Glimepiride (Amaryl)
- Glyburide (DiaBeta, Micronase)
- Glibenclamide
- Glicazide

In order for these drugs to have the most benefit, the patient must have a working pancreas and have Type 1 diabetes. Sulfonylureas boost the action of insulin at the cellular level and may directly reduce glucose secretion from the liver. They tend to be ineffective for illnesses that are characterized by a severe deficiency of insulin production. Sulfonylureas have first and second generation categories.

Side effects of sulfonylureas may include fluid retention, weight gain, and a slight increase in the risk of cardiovascular ailment, like a heart attack. You may also experience gastrointestinal symptoms and skin reactions. If you have delayed meals, no meals, or reduced intake of food and a minor increase in activity, hypoglycemia can result. Hospitalization may be required if complications occur, especially when the sulfonylurea is chlorpropamide.

Sulfonylureas interact negatively with other medications when consumed together. Specifically, severe hypoglycemia can occur. Examples of such medications that interact with sulfonylureas are sulfonamides, chloramphenicol, clofibrate, phenylbutazone, and bishydroxycoumarin.

A handful of sulfonylurea drugs have an indirect capacity to cause hyperglycemia. These agents include potassium-sparing diuretics like furosemide, corticosteroids, estrogen compounds, and diphenylhydantoin (Dilantin). Others can result in hypoglycemia, such as salicylates, propanolol, monoamine oxidase inhibitors, and pentamidine.

Second-generation sulfonylureas have the advantage of a shorter half-life and rapid filtration by the kidney and detoxification in the liver. These medications are safer for the elderly, who are more prone to recurring hypoglycemia.

Biguanides

Biguanides are yet another branch of diabetic drugs, and metformin (Glucophage) is among the most famous. Clearing the way for insulin's effect on receptor sites, these medications directly reduce sugar quantities in the circulatory system. They do not, however, have a pressing effect on the beta cells.

Together with a sulfonylureas, biguanides have the capacity to further reduce glucose.

Diabetics should be warned that lactic acidosis may result from biguanide use. Lactic acidosis is a serious complication, so close monitoring is required at the start of therapy or with dosage modifications.

Alpha Glucosidase Inhibitors

Examples of oral alpha glucosidase inhibitors are acarbose (Precose) and miglitol (Glyser), which are used in the management of Type 2 diabetes. These drugs act by delaying the absorption of glucose in the intestines and lead to a decreased postprandial blood glucose level. Due to reduced plasma glucose, hemoglobin A1C levels also are inhibited. Unlike sulfonylureas, acarbose, and miglitol, alpha glucosidase inhibitors do not have the possibility of producing unintended insulin increases. They can be utilized alone as a form of monotherapy.

Alpha glucosidase inhibitors should not be readily combined with sulfonylureas, thiazolidinediones, or meglitinides. When combined with sulfonylureas or meglitinides, hypoglycemia may result. If hypoglycemia does occur, the primary intervention should be glucose, not sucrose, since the latter is merely blocked.

One benefit of oral alpha glucosidase inhibitors is that they do not really need to be taken systematically, and they are relatively safer to use than many other diabetic treatments. They do have side effects, though, like diarrhea and flatulence (gas). These effects can be reduced by starting with a very low dose and increasing it a little bit at a time. Since acarbose and miglitol affect food absorption, they must be consumed immediately prior to consuming a meal.

Thiazolidinediones

Oral drugs that may be prescribed include thiazolidinediones like rosiglitazone (Avandia) and pioglitazone (Actos). Type 2 diabetics take these drugs along with insulin injections or when traditional sugar moderation is inadequate. Thiazolidinediones enhance the action of insulin at the receptor site without increasing the secretion of insulin from the beta cells. They also affect liver function, and in women they can cause resumption of ovulation, ultimately allowing pregnancy to occur.

Meglitinides

Repaglinide (Prandin) falls into a class of medications known as meglitinides. They enhance the release of insulin from pancreatic beta cells while decreasing glucose levels. The efficacy of meglitinides depends on the functioning of beta cells. Repaglinide should not be given to patients with Type 1 diabetes, since it acts rapidly but lasts for a very short amount of time.

Meglitinides should be taken prior to every meal to maintain the production of insulin as a reaction to consuming foods. They should be taken in conjunction with metformin. This is especially true for cases of hyperglycemia that are unmanageable with diet, exercise, or either metformin or repaglinide alone.

Primary side effects for meglitinides are far less serious or frequent compared to a sulfonylurea. This is due to the drug's reduced half-life.

Another meglitinide called nateglinide (Starlix) has a very quick onset and short duration. This should be taken in combination with meals, but not if a meal is skipped. There is some risk of becoming hypoglycemic if nateglinide is consumed on an empty stomach.

General Considerations When Using Oral Agents

Know that oral medications are not a substitute for other major treatment options. They are more like a supplement used in addition to diet and exercise. Once hyperglycemia occurs, or when there is infection, surgery, or trauma, oral medications may be discontinued temporarily in favor of the administration of insulin.

At some point, oral agents may not be enough to treat a person's condition, so the patient will have to receive insulin. Today, approximately half of those who take oral antidiabetic agents also take insulin. This is referred to as secondary failure. Primary failure means that blood sugar levels are abnormally high for a month following the use of a primary medication.

Due to the variation of drug interactions, multidosage oral medications may have a domino effect, so use them with care. Such medications containing varying mechanisms are very common today. A combination of oral agents and insulin is also recommended for those with Type 2 diabetes, but as for now, the effects still remain in question.

TREATMENT FOR DIABETIC NEUROPATHIC PAIN

Diabetic neuropathy is a serious matter for all of those who suffer from the pains of diabetes. Diabetes causes a lot of damage to its victims' nerves. Research carried out in this domain reveals that diabetic neuropathic pain is not only about nerve pain but about something more agonizing. A diabetic patient who suffers from diabetic neuropathic pain also experiences a peculiar wave of numbness in his or her feet. This kind of nerve pain is one of the common symptoms of diabetes, though it differs from person to person. For some diabetic patients, diabetic nerve pain is restricted to mild pain that can be endured and is not such a menace. For others, the pain is truly an agonizing, intolerable experience that is disabling. Proper and specific treatment is crucial for a total cure of diabetic neuropathic pain.

In order to tackle diabetic nerve pain head on, it is important to note that diabetic neuropathic pain is chiefly caused by high sugar levels and is experienced mostly at night.

A wide range of treatment procedures is available for getting rid of diabetic neuropathy. Before considering other aspects of treatment, it is better to consider some preventive measures. You may be aware of the golden maxim "Prevention is better than cure." If you really want to keep fit and stay away from diabetic neuropathic pain, try the following:

- Keep the existing sugar level in your body under control.
- Get rid of smoking forever.
- Stay physically active.
- Only eat nutritious and healthy foods.
- Stay away from junk food.
- Keep an eye out for bruises or swelling, or general red marks

Gaining complete relief from neuropathic pain is a hard-knock task, but different medications can be highly useful for this situation. These include the following:

- Tricylic antidepressants
- Topical anesthetics
- Codeines
- Antiseizure drugs
- Electrical stimulation of the nerves
- Narcotic pain relievers

Alpha lipolic acid is also prescribed for diabetes, since it is an antioxidant and may provide some minor relief.

TREATMENT FOR DIABETIC ABDOMINAL PAIN

Sadly, abdominal pain is a part of the lives of countless people throughout the world, both diabetics and nondiabetics alike. For nondiabetics, this type of pain is likely a sign of impending diabetes. In a study published in 2009 by the American Diabetes Association, experts claim that diabetes victims are likely to have experienced some form of abdominal pain; 75 percent of diabetes patients reported suffering from gastrointestinal concerns. Abdominal pain in diabetics usually manifests as gastroparesis, or delayed digestion. It can also be due to a yeast infection.

Whatever the cause, there are a variety of ways to address abdominal pain. If gastroparesis is at the root of one's abdominal pain, then medications such as cisapride and metclopropamide are prescribed. In the event that these drugs are not at your disposal, Amoxil or Zantac can curb neuropathic gastrointestinal pain to some extent. In addition, proper self-care has to be taken. Be strict in your diet in order to keep your sugar levels in check. Limited, controlled diets help the digestive process and hence halt abdominal pain caused by diabetes.

SUPPLEMENTARY GUIDELINES

In this chapter, we have taken a closer look at the care of patients who suffer from ailments associated with diabetes, and we have attempted to find appropriate treatments. Here are some additional instructions that will help diabetic patients heave a sigh of relief concerning crucial aspects like neuropathic pain, diabetic abdominal pain, and so on.

You should make it a point to learn about all the diabetic medications that lead to undesirable side effects. Anticoagulants, diuretics, corticosteroids, and oral contraceptives, among others, are drugs that fall into this category. Caution must be taken when using metformin for those with renal impairment or for those with a serum creatinine level greater than 1.4. Metformin is not advisable if you are at risk for kidney disease. It must be given for two days prior to any testing that makes use of a contrast agent, as these may cause lactic acidosis. Today, we have a combined form of metformin and sulfonylurea called Glucovance, which is available in an extended-release form that is much easier on the patient. You should understand the risk of hypoglycemia and keep in mind that heart disease patients are also vulnerable to it.

In the final analysis, tests of kidney function and renal screenings should be conducted frequently to make sure the urinary organs are performing up to par.

· *6* ·

Juvenile Diabetes

$\mathscr{W}$hen speaking of juvenile diabetes, we are referring to diabetes in children. What's more, many beliefs about juvenile diabetes of the past, such as the notion that children can only fall victim to Type 1 diabetes, have now been proven wrong.

DEALING WITH MISCONCEPTIONS

In the 1990s, an alarming trend took root: teen obesity. Children as young as ten were afflicted with juvenile diabetes, and since then this trend has reached epidemic proportions in the United States. Juvenile obesity cases have also risen in Europe, Australia, and Asia. Even the rate of children in Japan afflicted with obesity has reached levels on par with the United States. With all of these cases of obesity came an increase in juvenile diabetes.

This epidemic (which led to a rise in cases of juvenile Type 2 diabetes) is believed to have started in the 1980s, when experts noticed a distinct increase in the number of Type 2 diabetes cases among children of Native American descent. The number of cases rose steadily. Prior to 1994, juvenile Type 2 diabetes had only been found in 5 percent of youth who were newly diagnosed with diabetes, while the rest had Type 1 diabetes, which has always been more common among children. According to current estimates, approximately 45 percent or more of new cases of children with diabetes are Type 2.

In a study of Cincinnati children, cases of diabetes have increased during the last decade to ten times the previous level, from less than 1 case per 100,000 children in 1982 to 7.2 per 100,000 in 1994.

The juvenile diabetes epidemic has hit the minority community especially hard. According to a recent study, four out of every one thousand Native American teens are afflicted with diabetes. A similar study involving African American and Caucasian children aged ten to nineteen found that Type 2 diabetes accounted for 33 percent of all juvenile diabetes cases.

DIAGNOSING DIABETES IN YOUNGSTERS

The diabetes criteria for children are similar to those for adults: the fasting blood sugar (FBS) cutoff level is 126 mg/dL and above, while a postprandial blood sugar level of 200 mg/dL or above is considered diabetic.

Type 1 diabetes is a rather grave autoimmune disease caused by the failure of the pancreas to manufacture insulin. Usually this condition develops abruptly, and treatment sometimes involves the lifelong use of insulin and a growing need to follow a strict diet.

With Type 2 diabetes, the progress of the condition is not always simple and sudden. In the beginning stages, the pancreas gradually stops functioning and finally leads to a resistance to insulin. In children, Type 2 diabetes can almost always be prevented and even reversed through weight loss and a change in diet.

In the majority of cases, the physician has a difficult time determining whether the child is suffering from Type 1 or Type 2 diabetes because even those with Type 1 diabetes have a tendency to be overweight these days. About 24 percent of people are already overweight before manifesting any of the symptoms.

Being overweight can turn out to be a crucial factor in the development of Type 1 diabetes, since children weighing more than usual tend to have the disease at an earlier age compared to those who are not overweight. This is believed to be the reason behind the surprising statistics of Type 1 diabetes during the past decade.

If a child has Type 1 diabetes and is also obese, the child can have what is referred to as "double diabetes," which is insulin resistance due to obesity and, simultaneously, an inability of the liver to produce insulin due to the existence of Type 1 diabetes.

Adequate tests should be performed to detect diabetes early on, whatever type may be suspected. For example, in some cases of Type 2 diabetes, there may also be minimal production of insulin. If you have a history of Type 1 diabetes, you should monitor the health of your children. If you have a family history of Type 2 diabetes, attention should be focused on the prevention of obesity.

In the event of a positive Type 2 diagnosis in children, the same tests administered to adults are conducted: a glucose tolerance test, a fasting blood sugar level check, and a two-hour postprandial screening to identify the amount of insulin present in the pancreas.

THE SPOTLIGHT ON TYPE 1 DIABETES

Today, Type 1 diabetes is considered the most common severe chronic disease among children. Approximately 1 in 1,000 children in the United States below the age of nineteen have this ailment. Symptoms of Type 1 diabetes can include excessive thirst and hunger, frequent urination, sugar and ketones in the urine (glucosuria), and weight loss despite frequent eating. Children generally develop Type 1 diabetes between ten and twelve years of age for girls and between twelve and fourteen for boys. Type 1 diabetes can be hereditary, and the siblings of a Type 1 diabetic may be thirty times more at risk for contracting the illness compared to the general population. Meanwhile, the identical twin of someone with the disease has a 35 percent chance of contracting the disease.

Children with Type 1 diabetes may also display specific types of autoimmune antibodies, which is why there should be a test for the presence of C-peptide. This exam will reveal how much, if any, insulin is being produced by the pancreas. When insulin levels are extremely low, or no insulin being produced at all, we can assume the situation to be Type 1 diabetes.

TYPE 2 JUVENILE DIABETES

In Type 2 juvenile diabetes, the symptoms occur stepwise and are much less clear-cut. The basic indication is obesity, and approximately 80 percent of children with diabetes are extremely overweight or obese at the time of their diagnosis. Unlike those with Type 1 diabetes, children with Type 2 diabetes indicate very little in the way of weight loss. Usually they do not have increased thirst (polydipsia), excessive hunger, or frequent urination (polyuria). But a test of the urine usually discloses the presence of glucose.

Acanthosis nigricans is another common indicator of Type 2 diabetes, occurring in approximately 67 percent of patients with this type of insulin resistance. This condition includes patches of dark, velvety skin, generally on the neck, in the armpit region, or on other parts of the body where the skin rubs or comes to a fold. While this condition can occur at any age for other reasons, it can also suggest hyperinsulinemia, which is a precursor to diabetes.

Full-blown Type 2 diabetes can occur in children aged ten and up, to middle or late puberty. Insulin resistance gets worse as a person nears adolescence. Likewise, obese children have a natural tendency toward increases in insulin resistance. Children with at least one parent or immediate family member who became a diabetic during adulthood are more prone to the disease. Family history may also include past generations who suffered from either or both types of diabetes.

Ethnic origin also plays a role in contraction of the disease. African Americans, Hispanics, Asian Americans, Pacific Islanders, and Native Americans have a higher risk of this type of diabetes.

COMPLICATIONS OF TYPE 2 JUVENILE DIABETES

Children with Type 2 diabetes can be in great danger if their condition is not treated or managed well, and they can develop serious complications, as with Type 1 diabetes. A recent Swedish study on kidney disease in young adults with diabetes resulted in very distressing news. The experiment involved more than six hundred people from age fifteen to thirty-four who suffered from diabetes, with one group having Type 1 diabetes and others suffering from Type 2. Over a period of nine years, 5.6 percent of those with Type 1 diabetes and 16 percent of those with Type 2 diabetes developed kidney disease.

Similar studies looked at diabetic retinopathy, an eye disease connected to blindness when ignored and not treated as promptly as possible. Fifteen percent of those with Type 2 diabetes developed severe retinopathy, while only 5 percent of those with Type 1 got the severe form of the disease, with most of those with Type 1 getting a milder form.

These accounts describe how children with Type 2 diabetes can have serious complications from the disease. These accounts also remind us that younger age may be tied to a weaker ability to fight the symptoms. In contrast to most children who have diabetes, 80 percent of adults with Type 2 diabetes tend to only need insulin later in life.

Children with Type 2 diabetes are now given medications commonly prescribed to older people. Today, we can often find younger patients taking metformin (Glucophage) to retain proper blood sugar levels, in conjunction with other drugs used for combating high blood pressure, and sometimes with statin drugs used for high cholesterol.

TREATMENTS FOR DIABETIC CHILDREN

Treating a child with diabetes requires careful monitoring of the foods the child eats, focusing on healthy foods instead of the child's usual well-loved treats. When given controlled amounts of the right carbohydrates, children can lose weight and have more stable blood glucose levels. Discuss the proper diet with the child's doctor before proceeding with any changes in diet.

Note that treating diabetes in children may require more than one health care provider, especially if the child is taking medications. As blood sugar normalizes, it may be necessary to reduce dosages or even to eliminate dosages altogether to prevent hypoglycemia. Medications for controlling blood pressure and bloodstream lipids can be changed or slowly discontinued throughout the childhood years.

The goals and objectives of childhood diabetic therapies are similar to those of clinical measures for adults. First, doctors try to reduce carbohydrates to an appropriate level to control insulin and blood glucose levels. When blood sugar is stabilized, excessive feelings of hunger and cravings decrease. When glucose levels and impairments in insulin stabilize, lipid and blood pressure levels soon follow. As overall metabolism improves, there is a good chance that obesity can be reversed. Metabolic control by these procedures should be the ultimate objective in dealing with the juvenile diabetic's symptoms. It is advised that diabetic patients approaching puberty have their insulin and blood glucose levels supervised by a physician before attempting to change any treatment habits.

JUVENILE DIABETES AND EXERCISE

Besides controlling carbs, another preventative measure that should be highly regarded is exercise. For adults, the recommended workout time is at least a half hour per day. For children or young adults, exercise can take a different form. Any activity that keeps the child active is fine. Doctors advise keeping a record of the exercise performed every day of the week, just to monitor the progress of the child. This assures you that your child is exercising regularly. Keep an eye out for drops of blood during the course of or following physical exercise. This normally happens in children with Type 1 diabetes. Prior to exercise (approximately thirty minutes), the child should eat a protein-rich meal to help keep blood sugar at adequate levels during exercise.

Since young children have a propensity to be a bit defiant and extremely moody at times, parents need to constantly employ motivational strategies when shifting the child to a more specific diet regimen. Don't expect your child to respond positively to the changes right away, especially if you are not setting such a great example when it comes to healthy living yourself. Noticeable improvements should lead parents to make appropriate comments that will boost the child's confidence to accomplish more.

If there is a family history of obesity and a lack of participation in a healthy diet by the parents, a child may think, "What's the point?" If they don't see a tangible example of weight loss or a role model to look up to, they may follow the same patterns for eating and exercising that they see at home.

Always be mindful of the possible outcomes of not following a strict diet and exercise routine and falling back into the habits that bring about diabetes. You have to practice group activities in which kids with diabetes can learn to enjoy personal health management. Try to engage in healthier dietary options as well, so you can promote wellness throughout your family.

THE THIRD TYPE OF DIABETES

So far, we have been dealing with the two common types of diabetes: Type 1 and Type 2. There is also a third type that has recently been discovered called monogenic diabetes.

Monogenic diabetes differs from the previously known types, which are polygenic, or related to multiple genes. Monogenic diabetes surfaces as a result of the mutations of a single gene. This type of diabetes occurs in approximately 1 to 2 percent of the total cases of young people with diabetes. In certain instances, gene mutation occurs due to inherited traits and characteristics of family members. Gene alterations can also develop spontaneously, however, and through these mutations, the body suffers a reduced ability to develop insulin. As a result, monogenic diabetes is often mistaken as Type 1 diabetes.

Types of Monogenic Diabetes

The main types of monogenic diabetes include permanent neonatal diabetes (PND), transient neonatal diabetes (TND), and mature onset diabetes of the young (MODY). MODY is more common than TND or PND. While TND and PND primarily affect newborn babies and infants, MODY afflicts children and adolescents. The condition may be mild at first and not immediately diagnosed until the person reaches adulthood.

These variations may originate from different types of disease-causing genes. With this in mind, genetic testing may be used to diagnose the severest forms of childhood diabetes. If no genetic testing is carried out, the condition may be diagnosed and labeled as Type 1 or Type 2 diabetes.

Treatment can have an extremely positive effect on many patients, regardless of the type of diabetes. For others who experience milder symptoms, serious treatment may not be necessary.

SUPPORT SYSTEMS FOR CHILDREN WITH DIABETES

Parents should familiarize themselves with the proper treatment of juvenile diabetes. Above all, communication is vital. Parents should be aware of the importance of verbal interaction with the child patient, with doctors, and with other health care professionals. This keeps the relationship between parent and child close during a difficult time. When coping with a child with diabetes, you will realize how important it is to keep the lines of communication open in order to stay aware of any changes in mood or condition.

Try to make yourself available during the times when your loved one needs you. The young diabetic may be experiencing mood shifts that can be difficult to deal with, even for close relatives and friends. You may feel as if you want to give up, but you must continue in all your efforts against the diabetes epidemic.

Look for the light at the end of the tunnel. Are there things related to the condition that you might be missing? Probably. A young diabetic may sometimes hide discomfort behind mood swings, and it takes an extra effort by you to get him or her to verbalize feelings about diabetes. Stay open to changes in behavior that may not only affect health but can adversely affect relationships.

As mentioned earlier, it is vital that children emulate positive examples that parents display. Since the family is usually the main source of support, it is also important that juvenile diabetics gain the courage to face their struggles from their supportive parents and other members of the family.

DEALING WITH FRIENDS

When preteens or adolescents are diagnosed with diabetes, support from peers is forever important. Though some of their friends may understand the patient's condition and give him or her the approval and support needed, others may not recognize the severity of the situation.

According to research conducted by Dr. Alan Jacobson at Harvard's Joslin Diabetes Center, which involved children newly diagnosed with diabetes, 55 percent of the youngsters did not tell their friends they had diabetes, while 35 percent thought they would be liked more if they didn't have diabetes.

Gaining the support of their peers can help them manage their condition more efficiently and also boost their self-esteem. It is important for young diabetics to know that their friends and peers still accept them. This is why it is strongly advised that families and health care providers encourage children who have diabetes to be open about their condition, including with their peers. If peers are informed about the care measures related to diabetes, they might be able to assist the patient in coping with such a dreadful illness.

THE DIFFERENCES BETWEEN BOYS AND GIRLS

When comparing boys and girls with diabetes, we notice that most adolescent girls have a higher level of emotional support than boys. It has also been observed that girls were diagnosed and hospitalized with DKA (diabetic ketoacidosis) far more than boys. At this point, there is still no clear explanation as to why this occurs other than the obvious biological makeup of the individuals involved. There may be behavioral differences involving the amount of exercise or body image issues.

Fortunately, a good link exists between being athletic, having a good body image, and having well-controlled diabetes. Boys' general involvement in more physical activities may be one of the reasons why they have a better overall metabolic balance in their bodies.

Among young people without diabetes, adolescent girls tend to have more anxiety when compared to adolescent boys. Other factors, such as thought patterns and emotions in adolescents, may have a role in metabolic control.

Diabetes is easier to cope with when there is openness from family and friends. Diabetic patients can accept their condition with fewer reservations if there is a feeling that they will be able to manage their life with confidence and ease.

ON THE FINANCIAL ASPECTS OF JUVENILE DIABETES

Since having a child with diabetes will affect the entire family and will most likely require involvement from everyone around, the family must acknowledge the sacrifices it will make (money, time, patience, and more). Most importantly, make sure the young patient doesn't feel that he or she is a burden on the family. Consideration of the feelings of the young diabetic patient is important. It is vital that the patient feel that he or she is loved, that he or she is not a major disruption for the rest of the family, and that any shortcoming can be conquered with the family's support. A simple pat on the back of the loved one who may be in pain can go a long way toward relieving that pain.

Using creative stress management techniques and cutting costs for the better can keep the whole family intact during stressful times caused by juvenile diabetes. Are there insurance policies or medical supplies that are less expensive, ones that have the same quality and service as the major brands? Allow yourself to find the best, yet most economical, way to bear the burden your family is forced to take on.

When searching for healthier foods, take a look at food items that are less expensive than those processed by major brands but are still high quality. Since processed foods have been modified and have usually undergone many costly procedures, they have higher costs. Foods that are relatively unprocessed, like the fruits and vegetables that are recommended for diabetics, will often be cheaper and thus more accessible for children with juvenile diabetes. Of course buying in bulk is often cheaper than smaller packages.

You should also note the serving size you give to your diabetic child. Depending almost entirely on the form of diabetes, your child may have different nutritional needs with regard to quality and quantity. Does he or she have Type 1 or Type 2 diabetes? What about monogenic diabetes? Whichever type of diabetes your child has, you can propose a healthier diet for them after learning about the food items that are either necessary or that are bad for their health. You can also save money by only buying the foods that are specific to your child's needs.

PHASES OF THE JUVENILE DIABETES PATIENT'S LIFE

Diabetes and its related conditions change at different stages in the life of a child. You should remain informed about the development of diabetes in infants (birth to two years), toddlers or preschoolers (two to six years), school-age children (six to twelve years), adolescents (twelve to eighteen years), and young adults.

In addition to the biological and psychological changes in the child, there are social changes in the diabetic's journey through life. As a parent of a diabetic child, it is advisable to master the necessary skills and tasks to help him or her fight the disease. Try to learn the skills a child should master at a particular age, such as four. By this you can aid the child in doing what needs to be done.

You need a medical professional and other family members to give you support in caring for the child. A health care professional might recommend that you share with your child in the ups and downs that come with the disease, which will make the diabetic experience less troublesome for the child. It is also important that you be able to set healthy food choices for the juvenile diabetic.

In addition to the unusual situations that parenting a diabetic might present, there are the usual struggles that every child has to endure. These challenges might interfere with your relationship with the child and may also create problems in family relationships. However, you can help bridge the gap in these situations by using various coping mechanisms.

When caring for infants with diabetes, you may feel guilty about things that inflict pain, like the shots or certain testing requirements that are needed to detect the various manifestations of diabetes. You may find yourself second guessing about certain clinical procedures scheduled for the child. The young diabetic may grow tired of the feeling of being tested and monitored continually. Of course, you won't get the full cooperation of an infant, so you'll just have to employ certain tactics to make sure that the proper medical routines are followed. As a parent, you may be inclined to be overly cautious about certain medical procedures, but for them to be successful, your health care provider needs your full support.

Toddlers in general can be difficult to handle because of their occasional temper tantrums, which is due to the age of the child. Remember that children may be in tune with their parents' emotional state and are therefore likely to react to situations the same way his or her parents do. So, when explaining the different facts and procedures involved with diabetes to your son or daughter, try to be patient and calm. You can plan fun activities appropriate to the age of your child, and in doing so you can stimulate the imagination of the child so that he or she can accept a suitably healthy lifestyle. Juvenile diabetics should be able to eliminate or reduce some of their fear of things like medicinal injections and other treatments that may be initially tough to deal with.

When kids are introduced to educational and academic life beginning with kindergarten or pre-K, they get to meet new friends, so this period is important for showing the young patient that he or she is no different from his or her peers because of the illness.

Although being different isn't a bad thing, you can help the young patient feel that his or her differences really aren't negative qualities. Help them to regard their condition as a positive learning experience, allowing them to eventually acknowledge their condition with high self-esteem, thereby reassuring them that, even with the disease, they will always be special. If there is a need to have sugar levels checked while inside the classroom, the child can be taught not to feel ashamed or embarrassed while checking their diabetes. Be sure to involve children in the process as early as possible to keep their awareness and self-esteem in line.

When the child is finally able to do the necessary procedures by themselves, you can help by praising them for following the necessary therapeutic regimens. Failing to maintain recommended glucose levels should not make your child feel ashamed of telling you the results. The patient should easily gain control of life, making it easier for the family to deal with the juvenile diabetes.

When it comes to adolescents with diabetes, be aware of the *changes* in the youth's perspectives, experiences, and tendencies. Try to think of ways that can help the adolescent build confidence, and remember the struggle for self-awareness and the new responsibilities they must now handle in the midst of the typical emotional and physical turmoil experienced by teens. Even when you make the decision to let young people independently approach diabetes, remember that they are at a vulnerable and unpredictable stage of life. It is beneficial if you respect the moral, physical, emotional, spiritual, and social development of your adolescent son or daughter.

REINFORCEMENT MEASURES

According to psychologist Carol Dweck, it is better to praise a child's current actions rather than the outcome. Dweck emphasizes that giving due recognition for efforts that turn out to be successful is strongly recommended. This allows the child to engage in brand new or more challenging endeavors. When dealing with diabetes measurements in children, you can provide better encouragement and motivation if you look at the efforts the child has made rather than simply the glucose readings. Through this technique, you can have your child going as far as his or her confidence will allow.

In the long run, praising through words can be very helpful, as opposed to forceful actions that the child may grow numb to. However, the parent should not disregard external incentives that can be given to keep the child motivated.

If your reinforcement methods are verbal, the child will take the rewards more to heart, as he or she will feel that they are responsible for a healthier life for themselves. This will lead to a more mature physical and emotional state, rather than attenuating the child's feelings.

An experiment concerning the effects of parents' over-involvement in their children's lives (focusing on three-year-olds) was conducted by Dr. Kathleen Cain at Gettysburg College. The study found that mothers who consistently set high goals and overstress the child's mistakes cause their children to be ashamed for not achieving anything. These children soon become self-critical, self-conscious, and withdraw from others. A few children also displayed irregular behavior patterns and gave up much more easily on the tasks presented to them, possibly because they found it pointless to try to succeed if their parents were always complaining.

This study is a guide for all parents, but especially those of children with diabetes. It demonstrates that parents would do well to understand limits when it comes to their overall care for their children. Even if it seems natural for parents and other concerned individuals to direct and evaluate their children's actions and give constant feedback, it is wise to let children decide things for themselves. In a similar vein, children with diabetes can learn a lot on their own, deciding what works best for them in whatever possible ways are available. They can develop confidence that allows them to work toward their own development and personal enrichment.

Because of the numerous manifestations of diabetes, parents must also be able to let their children accept and cope with the physical and emotional cycles inherent to the disease. Don't let them feel that they are just there to please you by achieving goals; otherwise, they might turn these feelings into a premature excuse for isolation and distancing themselves from you.

REVERTING TO NORMAL

When we use the word *normal*, we mean that which pertains to the limits and disciplinary milestones gained by healthy children who don't suffer from diabetes. This process may entail educating yourself about the necessary strategies and knowledge needed for the particular age group of your child. You may be satisfied with your own parenting, but concerns with the diabetic child may force you to ask yourself, "What can I do in addition to what I'm already doing?" Finding out what is normal for your child's age group can help you determine if you are doing everything you can do.

JUVENILE DIABETES: THE LASTING EFFECTS

If we look at the problems that parents all over the world have in dealing with children who have diabetes, we observe that most aim at a balance between disciplinary measures, expectations, and permissiveness, while giving a certain amount of priority to the child's needs and pleasures.

The entire range of experiences that come with caring for a child with diabetes can make parents run through a range of emotions: compassion, love, concern, frustration, exasperation, and anger. In raising a young patient, there may be times when the parent will become furious with the child for not taking responsibility for their own well-being. If some parents encounter snags that interfere with managing their child, they might just feel like giving up altogether!

At the end of the day, proper disciplinary measures are the keys that permit parents to help their children manage their condition effectively.

WHAT TO DO DURING MEALTIMES

Parents often experience stress during mealtimes because they believe it's the right time and place to vent. In dealing with the dietary requirements of diabetic children, it is recommended that you practice the right household etiquette for all your children. You can take specific initiatives geared toward young diabetics and still exercise typical parenting rules. Set realistic parenting expectations even if your heart does not follow your mind. In so doing, you lead your child toward positive experiences during meals.

If your child has trouble focusing on their food at dinnertime, what can you do to help? Your normal instinct is to teach your child to like the food. When distractions like strawberry cheesecake appear on the breakfast table, ask the other members of the family to keep the child engaged in healthy eating habits. Try to make it a fun, yet healthy, dining experience.

PARENTS WORKING TOGETHER

You have to work with your husband or wife as a team to care for your diabetic child. Parents often wonder how to complement one another in the roles of mother and father. Both parents must learn how to take care of the tasks inherent in raising a child with diabetes. This can be extremely difficult at times, but it may turn out to be a rewarding experience after all.

In order to avoid emotional and physical exhaustion, keep your individual lifestyle fresh and engaging so that you can have meaningful experiences as your childrearing years go by. This is obviously impossible for the single parent of a child with diabetes, and occasionally the single parent may ask, "What can I do to help my son's condition if I'm single? I am alone and have no partner to help me out with my plight."

A single parent can try to look for a partner, which does not necessarily mean someone with whom the parent has an intimate relationship, but a person who is able to share the caretaking responsibilities for a juvenile diabetic. This could easily be the grandmother of your child. Both of you can work together and be partners while caring for the child who has diabetes.

Looking after the youngster can involve painful and heartbreaking experiences, so it is wise to remember the child's needs and to remember the strategies that are needed to raise a healthy child. There may be times when one or both parents may feel like there is no hope for fighting off the disease. They simply go ahead and accept that this is their lot in life, their cross to bear.

Help from a partner can get a parent past these feelings. If the mother is able to always keep the child's blood sugar level down, but the father turns out to be a failure in this regard, the parents might clash over the issue. The father might feel depressed if something unfortunate happens to the child, while the mother may likewise feel guilty because she wasn't the one taking responsibility.

Guilt and conflict over responsibility could make matters worse for the young patient. There has to be the realization that everyone has certain skills for meeting the needs of the young patient. For instance, if the father takes responsibility for monitoring blood sugar levels, then he will also be in control of his overall attitude toward the patient and the disease, and thus the diabetes can be managed more effectively.

A father who has plenty of time to give to the child will therefore have a better understanding of the skills needed to manage the disease. In contrast, when the father has limited involvement in the management of the disease, he will most likely have a difficult time dealing with situations requiring intensive treatment.

Of course, the child may have his or her own preferences when it comes to administering care. The child may want to have his mother take care of him instead of his father. Depending on the relationship between the two parents, this could affect the overall care of the child. The father may grow envious of the attention the child gives to the mother. On the other hand, there may be competitive feelings between the two spouses, especially when both of them are vying for the child's attention.

By all means, this does not imply that the mother or father is the better parent. If the parents of the patient are living together, they will both have an equal opportunity to assist their child in coping with the disease. The patient benefits when a parent gets a chance to express his or her thoughts and become more open to the family. For instance, the father can acknowledge any of his own frailties in the matter and seek help from his spouse to better handle the dilemma, and the mother can concurrently acknowledge that she can help her husband and child by being supportive of both of them. Opportunities that allow both parents to take care of the patient equally should always be sought.

When dealing with juvenile diabetes, it is important to come up with techniques in which everyone in the family can work together and attain the goal of combating the disease, particularly with all of the difficulties along the way. As children who have not yet reached maturity, they require a certain amount of guidance, which should come especially from parents and relatives. Caretakers of diabetic children should therefore see to it that they acquire a vast amount of knowledge and understanding of what the child might go through. Diabetic children may not always be able to express their feelings, but with your compassion, their symptoms can be addressed appropriately.

Part Three

OTHER MANIFESTATIONS

· 7 ·

Diabetes and Mental Health

$\mathscr{D}$iabetes has a tremendous impact on a patient's mental health. Besides the physical manifestations and complications affecting the heart, kidneys, liver, eyes, nerves, and other organs, associated shifts in emotions can personally affect the diabetic and his or her family.

Psychological consequences of diabetes are always just around the corner, so it is essential to stay focused in tackling the disease. A diabetic can lack disciplinary routines to the extent that family members get anxious and concerned about inadequacies in their efforts to help the diabetic. A diabetic's life experience as a whole can thereby lead to a lack of self-esteem and concern about ruined relationships.

The diabetic in question, or a next of kin, or someone who cares about diabetes has the capacity to turn the tide and make living with diabetes easier and safer. It takes time and commitment, but with the use of support mechanisms, the mental health of a diabetic individual can be positive in the long run.

MENTAL HEALTH COMPLICATIONS LINKED WITH DIABETES

Stress is a possible effect of diabetes, both to the sufferer and to family members. Unexpected challenges and various complications may arise from symptoms and gradually lead to unhealthy thoughts and emotional strife.

Damaged Self-Esteem

One complication that seems to go unrecognized in diabetics is the turn of emotions. When self-esteem decreases, the patient's mind may become preoccupied with anxiety and personal dilemmas, and may succumb to a lack of self-consciousness.

Considerations pertaining to diet, lifestyle, and exercise may instill mental feelings of apprehension upon having to abandon certain bad habits. To combat this, there must be a willingness to succeed in the battle against diabetes. A patient should be assisted against distress caused by the disease and in making transitions easy despite having to alter a few personal habits every now and then. As always, someone affected by diabetes may choose to be proactive and approach their situation in a positive way that allows them more control over their mental and physical health.

Your self-esteem has various effects on your lifestyle, including your job, marriage, parenting, and other aspects vital to your happiness and physical health. With the physical effects of diabetes, you may seriously think to yourself, "Why has this happened to me? Will I ever be without the pain I am going through? I feel that I am a burden on my family, and I can't help feeling this way."

With modern tools for treating and managing diabetes, such as insulin pumps and blood glucose monitors, some patients tend to be more conscious about their health because of the accessibility and convenience of these procedures. Patients who do not have access to such treatment tools, or who cannot use such devices, or who are limited in their movement, may set themselves apart from other diabetics who live much differently. Some patients may also feel deprived from the life they once enjoyed and may deny themselves pleasure because of their condition.

If you think you are alone in this battle, think again! There are definitely more ways to experience life other than the usual exploits that are now part of your daily routine. People will have their opinions, but ultimately it is you, the patient, who are in control of your life. Even if your health care professional can assist you with achieving your health goals, you still have the ability to work toward your own well-being. You can also gain knowledge of your situation and your health. In that respect, you should continue to work according to your own rules and impulses, but with guidance from medical professionals.

Fear

Fear is another complication of diabetes related to mental health and emotions. Fear signals that you may not be doing things to help yourself, which can lead to negative thinking. Fear can manifest itself in your actions. This may hinder you from asking questions of others, which consequently gives you a lack of control.

Having such fears may also deprive you of various necessities of health that can be enjoyed. The solution is to face these obstacles head on. Fear indirectly suggests that a patient may not be properly combating their diabetic symptoms.

Practice communicating with your doctor or health care professional to manage your diabetes. If you develop a sense of fear of your situation, talk to your doctor. Diabetes can be an extremely unpredictable disease, but through proper communication with friends and family, you will be well equipped to win the battle.

Loneliness

Due to the periodic buildup of the complications and manifestations of diabetes, there may be a point when the diabetic feels like giving up. It all boils down to the attitude you have with respect to the mental experiences you are going through as a diabetic. Even though people may tell you there is no known cure for diabetes, it is no reason to quit caring entirely.

As you know, various support systems are available for diabetics. In most cases it just takes a simple call or visit to the right place to help you out with any mental difficulties you may have, including loneliness.

Grief

If you are a diabetic, it is natural to grieve, but you must avoid feeling sorry for yourself. If you look at the natural process of grieving, you will learn that from denial, in which a person does not accept the reality of the situation, the affected person can easily proceed to anger.

When angry, the diabetic may become rebellious against the situation. This may be a natural response, as there may not be any possible way to express one's feelings without the use of negative thoughts and ideas, including excessive grief.

The next stage in grieving is bargaining. At this point, one may feel like making a deal with the gods that be, saying, "If you take away my diabetes, I will be a better parent, a better learner, and a much better human being."

Bargaining is followed by depression. There is a tendency for diabetics (especially those in the terminal stages of the disease) to be depressed. At times, the depression may get more uncontrollable, leading to feelings of hopelessness and even suicidal impulses.

The last stage of grief is acceptance. After all that has happened, there will soon come a time when the person has already accepted fate and is ready to face anything that may come along. The diabetic may come to believe that everything is actually within reach. There is no point of drowning in loneliness and despair in the midst of commitment and discipline to overcome the disease. When choosing health care providers, it is highly recommended that you have compassionate physicians and other health care professionals with a deep commitment for providing genuine services to those in need.

DEPRESSION

According to demographic and psychographic studies conducted on diabetic patients, females are twice as prone to depression as males. Fewer men seek treatment for a depressive state of mind. This is thought to be a result of the macho image that many men try to portray. They think that being a man requires both silence and strength during pain.

Clinical depression, however, must not be left unacknowledged and ignored. The improvement of one's state of mind can make one better able to cope with certain stresses, and thus enable one to manage diabetes more effectively.

Sadly, people are overconfident that they can fix depression themselves and thus decide not to seek professional help. They don't realize that learning the right methods from health care professionals is in fact one of the most effective techniques for achieving good health.

Given the prevalence of diabetes, the most common measure taken to combat diabetes-related depression is probably self-help. This can take the form of reading texts (such as this book), keeping oneself occupied with worthwhile activities, mentally challenging any negative thoughts that come to mind, practicing positive thinking, and helping others in similar situations. It is equally important that you become familiar with the signs of depression so that you can prevent it or seek help if you become seriously depressed.

Having three or more of the following symptoms for at least two weeks indicates that it is time to seek help for depression.

- Shifts in sleep patterns, such as oversleeping or insomnia
- Weight loss or weight gain
- Constant feelings of sadness
- Difficulty concentrating
- Feelings of nervousness or anxiety during times of relaxation
- Feelings of guilt or thoughts of being a burden to others
- Feeling hopeless or worthless
- Thoughts of suicide

Working Hard to Combat Depression

Being told to lose weight or to face daily insulin injections can be devastating, but there is no sense in avoiding treatments simply because you are frustrated or ashamed, or to believe that all of your mental problems will vanish by tossing out the extra pounds.

When surrounded by such feelings, you might have the tendency to hide from your family members and health care providers, since you don't want them to know about your situation and your vulnerability.

When depression takes shape, you could decide to endure it and to consider it a part of life that will soon pass, but this can make your condition even worse. Don't drown your emotions with alcohol, drugs, or food, believing that doing so will relieve all your symptoms. Whichever technique for dealing with depression you take advantage of, remember that these techniques are most effective when carried out under the guidance of a health care professional.

EATING DISORDERS

Another common complication of diabetes is eating disorders. To avoid eating disorders, get an idea of how good or bad your condition is before taking dietary measures.

There are complications that occur with diabetes that may make you think you are way too thin for your height and weight, or perhaps that you are obese based on your BMI. Furthermore, your blood sugar levels may be elevated, thus requiring various medications. If left untreated, complications can surface, including coma and even death.

When learning about diabetes, you might come to realize that correct food intake is important, and depression can cause you to eat more. Your family members and health care professionals should be aware of certain of your habits, including those that are dietary. Eating disorders can morph into an obsession to get dangerously thin. Unfortunately, body image, shame, and secrecy become major issues rooted in being powerless, depressed, anxious, lonely, angry, or obsessive.

Anorexia

Anorexia is an eating disorder characterized by a constant longing to become excessively thin. People with anorexia want to lose weight even though they are already dangerously slim. Anorexics have a disturbed body image, diminished menstrual periods, and a loss of sexual interest. To lose weight, they fast, diet, and exercise in the absence of external forces like peer pressure. Their moods are disturbed because they are in a state of semistarvation. At first, losing weight may be a technique for taking control or feeling good, but over time, the anorexic behavior turns into a mental fixation on weight loss and starvation.

Bulimia

The diabetic occasionally yearns to lose weight but tends to overeat as well. In the end, he or she becomes regretful and purges undigested food later in the day. Bulimia involves episodes of binge eating, in which the person takes in amounts of food beyond what is typically capable of being ingested. This food is then expelled through vomiting.

Simply put, binging involves a lack of control in appetite, metabolism, and diet. It is then followed by schemes to overly restrict one's lifestyle and engage in too much exercise.

If you happen to be bulimic, avoid reducing or eliminating your insulin medications, since this may lead to DKA (diabetic ketoacidosis) or hyperosmolar coma. Bulimia is different from anorexia in that patients are more aware of the fact that what they are doing is very unhealthy. Thus these individuals are more apt to participate in psychological therapy than sufferers from anorexia.

Binge Eating

Affecting approximately 20 percent of those who are obese, binge eating is considered an increasingly rampant mental and physical issue. Binge eaters don't really want to lose weight, and they avoid the purge cycle found in bulimia. They do three or more of the following: eating fast, eating excessively even though they are not hungry, eating until they are full, eating alone due to consciousness of the high amount of food being eaten, and feeling distressed about eating. The latter often gives way to depression and guilt, and the affected diabetic doesn't mind gaining any weight, given the circumstances. These binging episodes generally take place a minimum of two days a week and last for around six months at a time.

Research has indicated a strong relationship between binge eating, dissatisfaction with weight, poor compliance with diabetes care measures, and levels of depression. Those who are more likely to suffer from depressive episodes due to binge eating include a higher proportion of elderly people and males, and an equal rate of African Americans and Caucasian Americans. A mental health professional can guide someone with these specific problems.

Insulin Manipulation

Another problem associated with diabetics is insulin manipulation. This is the frequent use of insulin to regulate food consumption. Insulin manipulation afflicts a large number of people who have diabetes. The problem stems from fears of gaining weight or recurring thoughts of the possibility of hypoglycemia. According to medical research, 31 percent of people dispose of their insulin after using the recommended dosage. However, 8 percent take insulin excessively, thereby leading to complications that could be severe. Problems that could arise include hypoglycemia and death.

Dealing with Eating Disorders

Having diabetes and eating disorders concurrently raises hemoglobin and induces hypoglycemia due to purging or restriction of food. It also brings on episodes of ketoacidosis. Eating disorders can therefore cause serious damage to the health of diabetics. Hence, there need to be effective, practical education measures; therapeutic regimens that involve individual, marital, and group contributions; and even antidepressants and antianxiety agents. Exercise and counseling about nutrition are vital, too.

Following the diagnosis of a diabetic's eating disorder, both the individual and his or her family members could find themselves dealing with feelings of self-doubt, blame, guilt, resentment, and anger.

With the recommendations from an endocrinologist or diabetologist, there may be a way around all of the painstaking measures required to overcome these mental symptoms. In practice, the guidelines below should be followed as much as possible:

- Balancing privacy with social life
- Getting through conflict
- Emphasizing true beauty that does not depend on weight
- Focusing on feelings, not food
- Making mealtimes pleasant
- Doing away with aggressive or controlling food behaviors
- Discussing situations that may be uncomfortable (such as dining out in restaurants)
- Continuing to perform activities that seem worthwhile and pleasurable to the diabetic

Among these considerations, the one with the highest importance is focusing on feelings, not food. If you don't practice good thinking and feeling, you might develop unhealthy coping behaviors.

THE MENTAL HEALTH PROS

Besides members of the medical team discussed in the previous chapter, we should take a good look at the expertise of *mental* health care professionals. Being experts in psychology, these professionals will help you to learn about your emotions, boost your self-confidence, and guide you toward fulfilling self-motivation. They can also help you with behavioral changes.

To take the best advantage of available services, you should cooperate and allow mental health professionals to utilize the psychological mechanisms needed to bring forth good results in your treatment. Just like you, they have weaknesses that may hinder their work if presented with unnecessary challenges. Have a win-win relationship with your mental health care professional by following their recommendations and course of treatment. The goal is simply to take your best shot in working for your own mental wellness.

Stress Related to Prediabetes

Patients who suffer from prediabetes experience stress too, which can then lead to diabetes itself, since severe stress raises the level of blood sugar. Together with the severe stress caused by a specific illness, "counter-regulatory" hormones may also be activated. These hormones work to ensure that there are lots of sugars to help your body react against intense moments. They also allow the liver to produce sugar and to make the body more resistant to insulin's ability to decrease the levels of blood glucose.

Though stress itself cannot cause prediabetes in a person who is not at risk, it can affect a person's behavior, and the levels of blood sugar, in various ways. It is advisable to limit stress in your daily life whenever you can. Also take note of how you react to daily stressors and take charge of your own feelings. For many patients, food is somewhat like an imaginary cradle when they are stressed. Others just go to sleep or feel so overwhelmed that they hide from society because they think they will be misunderstood. A diabetes prevention program can help patients develop good habits for their own wellness and avoid stress.

Beyond this, various techniques are available to help diabetics conquer stress. Participate in deep breathing exercises. Proper inhalation and expiration (which you may not be doing right now) can do wonders for your mental health. When you engage in proper breathing, you can relieve yourself of a lot of tension.

Yoga is also strongly encouraged for the stressed-out diabetic. You will also do well if you balance yoga with meditation, the end result of which is a refreshed mind. It even helps a blurred mind to become clearer.

Have you ever thought about getting a professional massage? By participating in such stress-reducing activities, you can get ideas about other antistress techniques. More strategies will be presented in chapter 11, when we tackle motivational methods useful for diabetes patients.

A FRIED BRAIN: DIABETES AND BRAIN FUNCTION

According to a research study by Dr. Sophie Yeung of the University of Alberta, mild diabetes may cause the slowing of brain function. While not considered a major cognitive defect, reduced brain activity, based on the study, begins during the early phase of Type 2 diabetes. Luckily for those with mild to moderate diabetes, this deterioration is not severe. The study was conducted on 570 adults aged fifty-three to ninety, 41 of whom had the relatively mild type of diabetes, with mental screenings every three years. As well, Dr. Roger Dixon of the University of Alberta believes that past studies indicate that diabetes ultimately results in mental deterioration.

Unsurprisingly, most diabetics have healthy reaction times and perceptual speeds. They are, however, slower at carrying out tasks requiring fast and precise processing of new information consisting of words. These defects involve speed, not verbal fluency. Dixon also mentions that using proper management at the earliest possible time can prevent these manifestations.

Even if these findings are to be believed, note that they do not suggest any medical correlation between age and potentially *major* psychological decline.

THE RELATIONSHIP OF AMPUTATION TO
MENTAL HEALTH IN DIABETICS

Based on a study performed on American veterans with diabetes, depleted mental functioning has an unsafe effect on diabetics' mental well-being and is proportional to a higher risk of having amputations.

Dr. Chin-Lin Tseng led the project at the Veteran Administration's New Jersey Health Care System in East Orange, New Jersey. The team found that mental functioning must be assessed in relation to other risk factors for major amputation.

Tseng analyzed 115,000 diabetes patients who received medical care from Veterans Health Administration clinics between 1998 and 2000; the patients were asked questions about their mental health, and data were collected regarding amputations.

For patients with below-average mental functioning, the total rate of major amputation turned out to be 0.5 percent, and for those with above-average mental functioning it was 0.3 percent. In addition, those with the highest level of mental functioning had an amputation rate of only 0.2 percent.

PSYCHOTIC ILLNESSES AND DIABETES

Individuals with psychosis who are on new antipsychotic medications may have an elevated risk of developing diabetes and related metabolic diseases. It has also been found that those with diabetes are twice as likely to have depression as nondiabetics.

Numerous factors bring about the susceptibility of long-term mental patients to diabetes and cardiovascular disorders, including suboptimal access to medical services, frequent smoking, poor diet, a sedentary lifestyle, and obesity.

Medical research is currently focused on a possible link between antipsychotic medications and diabetes, just as there are connections between diabetes and depression. Health professionals must be concerned with ensuring care for the mental, emotional, *and* physical health of their diabetic patients. In doing so, doctors will be demonstrating quality and complete care for those they have sworn to protect and care for whenever needed. The risk of such illnesses comes about as a result of disorganized lifestyles, antipsychotic medications, and pathophysiological effects that can only be discovered through intensive studies on the inner workings of the brain in response to disease.

At the same time, medical practitioners have to take note of a range of antipsychotic drugs that have different effects, such as hyperglycemia, weight gain, and other disturbances in metabolism. There must be careful consideration of the drugs prescribed to someone, especially drugs prescribed for their antipsychotic effects.

As only a few experiments have indicated a relationship between diabetes and antipsychotic medications, there is a call for further research to accurately describe such effects and to find improved treatment options for diabetes and related disorders.

DIABETES IN RELATION TO SCHIZOPHRENIA

Various reports indicate a relationship between diabetes and psychiatric disorders. However, these studies generally do not take age, gender, family history, race, and obesity into consideration. They also ignore important elements like the timing and details of drug administration.

Newer schizophrenia medications may interfere with control of hyperglycemia by altering blood glucose levels, as contrasted with older medications such as risperidone. Other differences in the effects of newer and older drugs may be due to diabetics having been tested prior to or after taking the medications. Or they could be due to the nature of the diagnostic exam used to detect diabetes in the first place.

To shed light on the relationship between diabetes and schizophrenia, we should reflect on research demonstrating that 15 percent of those with schizophrenia also have diabetes, as compared to 3 percent of the general population. Similarly, older diabetic populations and those of African American descent are also at higher risk for acquiring such mental illness.

Different varieties of drugs have already been developed to combat schizophrenia and other psychiatric disorders. Antipsychotic medications are categorized into first and second generation, or *typical* and *atypical*. Second-generation drugs are relatively new, having been in use for twenty years or less. They are also known to have less severe side effects, thus being favored by the majority of diabetes management professionals.

In particular, drugs that inhibit the secretion of insulin include thiazide diuretics, calcium channel antagonists, phenytoin, pentamidine, and cyclosporin A. As well, streptozocin results in the destruction of beta cells.

As for sympathetic nervous system stimulation, alpha and beta agonists and antagonists and xanthenes are the real drugs to think about. Corticosteroids, oral contraceptive pills, and anabolic steroids cause impaired insulin action. The effects of nalidixic acid, rifampicin, isoniazid, and phenothiazines are still not entirely known.

STRESS LEVELS

Just as there are tools for measuring intelligence and emotion, there are handy devices that provide us with a stress quotient (SQ). These machines enable you to obtain a more tangible type of data for testing one's ability to handle stress.

Personal Stress Monitors

You should perform a self-check to determine your stress levels each day, most especially during the early morning when you wake up and in the evening just before you go to sleep. When you first wake up, what do you think of immediately? Do you feel angry, upset, or worried? Jot these thoughts down and make sure you address them as soon as you wake up if possible. Try to consider the worst possible scenario. Plan alternative possible approaches when faced with uncertain circumstances. Try noting three things you are thankful for in the midst of all the stress you go through.

Prior to falling asleep, reflect on your day with thoughts of thankfulness. Also write down the things you have completed or will accomplish soon, making a commitment that you will deal with these things the following day. You cannot expect to finish all of your weekly tasks in one day, or to finish an assignment that usually takes a year in a month. Just do your best to accomplish what you need to do to be successful in your endeavors, leading a stress-free day. At night, the unconscious mind will generally tap various resources to help you come up with plans and solve problems.

Relationship Focus

Again, at some point after waking up or before going to bed, reflect on the relationships that encompass the large part of your life. Do you have anything to say or do that is not done yet? If there are things like this, when is the best time to do or say these things? Well, the sooner it happens, the better. You also need to note that positive thinking works like magic. Therefore, the key to stress reduction in relationships includes constant communication and honesty.

Reduce the Level of Stress

Meditation and relaxation can definitely help during a time of stress. They give resilience to the body and will serve you well. Try to say a prayer repeatedly in your mind, soothing yourself with every word that flows from the prayer and calming the space within. Don't hurry when doing this. Meditate and reflect fervently, mentally focusing on the fact that you are handling your mind with ease and that you are filled with good thoughts. Gracious emotions and heavenly thoughts are what we all really wish would surround us at all times. When you meditate, you are really preparing yourself to be focused and strong enough to employ creative techniques to handle the stresses and mental challenges that you face.

POSITIVE REFRAMING

The processes involved in thinking, speaking, and communicating with oneself and others are part of the psychological toolbox that can promote positive interventions when stressed by the complications of diabetes.

Let's dig deeper into positive reframing. It is all about changing the way you see things. With positive reframing, you will be able to look at something that others might consider devastating as something positive that is an opportunity for you to grow psychologically. You are just moving outside of the box, realizing that the overall picture is a lot bigger when you don't concentrate only on things seen with the naked eye. Consequently, you are exposing yourself to the other side of the story. Try to consider what might really be happening instead of shunning the very facts that are being repeatedly pushed toward you.

Imagine your spouse yelling, "You are doing nothing to help yourself." Your response might be to think that your spouse does not love you or completely understand you. Perhaps he or she always criticizes you, and you have a problem with that. First try to recognize the source of the conflict. Then try to continue with thoughts that allow you to feel more positively. The truth is that your spouse is just as concerned about your diabetes as you are, if not more so. Try not to think about the fact that she is yelling at you. At the back of your mind, you know that she is just worried and fearful since she loves you. You don't have to transmit your anger back at her simply because you hope she'll stop behaving the way she does.

In the psychological field, therapeutic communication is really of great importance. This is because when health care providers are interacting with their patients, they should make sure they are not communicating their biases or indulging in their personal urges to say something without knowing the entire story. Furthermore, for a patient who is experiencing all the stress that goes with diabetes, caretakers should practice therapeutic communication. This entails habitual practice! As you develop an understanding of the particular reasons a certain situation has occurred, you give yourself a chance to reflect and understand what needs to be done.

COPING TECHNIQUES FOR DIABETICS

When a person discovers that he or she suffers from diabetes, there will be a combination of emotions that fill the person's thoughts, feelings, and actions. If you are a diabetic, or the significant other of a diabetic, are your coping mechanisms healthy? You may have been using different methods to cope with different situations, but how can you improve your reactions to all such situations?

Responses to the complications of diabetes are developed from inner thoughts. There are coping techniques that exist as a natural part of who a person is. Sometimes these reactions last for only a short time, while some last for a very long time. For instance, as a diabetic, you may be fearful and self-conscious whenever people see you experiencing the symptoms of hypoglycemia. You may in due course develop a coping strategy, like preventing hypoglycemia by allowing your blood sugar level to remain high. This strategy may bring you short-term relief. But you will still have to bear the unpleasant effects this strategy will have on you in the long run. You will soon begin to experience excessive thirst, irritability, and too much urination. This is what we call an avoidant behavior.

Furthermore, you may try other techniques, like using drugs, engaging in sexual activities, drinking liquor, and eating more frequently than usual to cope with stress. These reactions may have negative outcomes once you experience the harmful results that such behavior can bring about.

To avoid such maladaptive forms of behavior, you should begin by honestly assessing the situation, admitting to yourself that you have a problem, and committing yourself to combating the problem with the best solution there is. Such solutions may include keeping a daily journal, using humor, telling stories related to the situation (a form of venting), and seeking social support, which can come from friends, family members, and other sources. All of these strategies will help you to examine your feelings closely enough that you can handle the stressful aspects of your life.

Diabetics may attempt to shift their thoughts and behaviors if difficulties arise. In some situations, negative behavior can be reversed and turned into positive behavior. For instance, you might be drinking too much because you feel this is a way of getting out of the mess you are in. To distract yourself from this behavior, you might come up with an enjoyable hobby or interest, thereby allowing you to engage in more worthwhile activities that can keep you occupied and functioning better. In doing so, you are promoting rational thoughts and allowing them to flow from your mind, thus enabling you to stay on the go with the daily pressures in life.

At times, indulging in charitable actions does the trick. Try to make the best out of your condition by developing techniques for being of service to others. As you may already know, a sense of fulfillment can be achieved by performing selfless actions, which allow you to bring out your own goodness. This is referred to as altruism.

If you are ever looking for a place where altruism really exists in the world today, try looking into local support groups. As volunteers and others listen and help those who are willing to make a change for their own wellness, those who need help end up feeling mentally refreshed and confident. They begin to see themselves in a different light. They acknowledge that they are powerful and have the capacity to work for their own mental health.

CHALLENGING YOU

Thoughts and feelings often need to be challenged, and sometimes this requires you to let go of something you thought you could never do without. Examples include junk food and late night TV. As you detach yourself from such things, try to envision yourself as your own personal life coach. The point here is to see yourself in a different way.

Negative and potentially damaging thoughts may be automatic and beyond human control, but we can still create resistance to these ruminations. Negativity, if addressed properly, can be converted to positivity. This may require very little effort at times, but at other times, deeper analysis may be required.

Distinct patterns of negativity are easily recognized by those around you. If you already know that you have these negative patterns and you attempt to address them accordingly, you are not only protecting yourself mentally, but you are gaining further trust from your peers. It may also boost your confidence as far as dealing with the mental aspects of diabetes.

The All-or-Nothing Pattern

In the all-or-nothing pattern of thinking, you get these feelings that are simply caught between good or bad, black or white. You seem to have no space for the gray portions of reality. The all-or-nothing pattern of thinking suggests that if something isn't good, then it must be utterly bad, and hence you are getting yourself into a whole lot of trouble.

Just look at this scenario: As a diabetic, you need to be on a restricted diet. Your doctor may have already instructed you to avoid eating sweets, but you are still tempted and eat your favorite pastries, which is really a no-no. With an all-or-nothing pattern of thinking, you might come to think that you are a bad person.

Never or Always

For some diabetics, everything must be perfect. The person with this kind of thought pattern usually has "shoulds" and "musts." Such a person must believe that things are perfect, or else depression will surface. This attitude is not exactly the best attitude, because it just brings about more inner turmoil.

Selected Negativity

With this pattern of thought, you tend to focus only on the negative aspects of a situation. You keep your eyes mainly on the problem. You consider only what you see with the X on it, instead of the different sides of the situation. When you adopt such a pattern of thinking, you may end up creating an inaccurate perception of reality.

Emotional Focus

This pattern of thinking focuses on the feelings experienced in a particular situation. When a diabetic is feeling down, he or she may sadly accept his or her fate and come to believe that depression is really the main purpose of life, without actually addressing the problem face to face.

In conclusion, bear in mind that positive thinking and recognizing depressive behaviors can help all patients mentally defeat their diabetes.

· 8 ·

Diabetes and Heart Health

$\mathscr{H}$eart disease is alarming when it becomes part of a diabetic's life. Note this statistic: approximately 75 percent of diabetics die of heart problems.

The deteriorating state of health known as metabolic syndrome leads to unrestrained plaques that cause narrowing of the arteries and reduction of blood flow to the heart. If left unchecked, this can also lead to arterial blockage, which causes heart attacks. Half of those who experience a heart attack will die within the first hour, and many won't even make it to the hospital. Even if they survive the attack, their heart muscles will never be able to work the same way.

THE UNRULY MAGIC OF THE HEART

When diabetes and heart disease work together, there can be a deadly outcome. In fact, having diabetes leads to a higher risk of heart attack.

Once you have diabetes, you are at risk for heart disease, even though you might not have previously had it. This is because when a person develops diabetes, his or her blood vessels are gradually damaged, often resulting in heart disease. As long as you have the capacity to control your diet, you also possess the power to manage your own health as a diabetic. You *can* come to grips with heart disease if you take the necessary steps to reduce the risks.

Aside from monitoring your blood sugar and blood pressure levels, you should also consider your lipids, which are the fats and cholesterol circulating around inside of you. If you are considering ways to decrease your cholesterol levels, you might not want to go for conventional means of treatment, like taking medication, right off the bat. You should learn early on about the root causes of the problem and treat them first.

If you already have diabetes or think you might be heading for it, know that your risk is greater for heart disease. In fact, according to a screening of 118,000 men and women in Harvard's Nurses' Health Study, the risk of developing diabetes is approximately four times as high if you have a heart problem. Researchers in this study observed the participants for twenty years. Yes, *twenty* years!

At the beginning of the study, 1,500 patients had diabetes, while about 390 had a history of heart disease. In the two decades of the study, at least 6,000 more got diabetes, and 2,500 were newly diagnosed with coronary heart disease. Through this study, researchers discovered that women who have diabetes and prior heart disease are twenty times more likely to die from cardiovascular diseases, such as stroke, and twenty-five times more likely to die from coronary heart disease.

The findings don't just apply to women. Middle-aged nondiabetic men with high levels of glucose are at a higher risk for death, not just from heart disease, but from all other causes as well. This was learned from intensive studies published in Australia, where again thousands of participants were examined and observed over the course of many years. Among the participants in these studies, patients exceeding the upper 20 percent of healthy glucose levels had a risk of heart disease 1.6 times higher than those with sugar amounts in the lower 80 percent of preferred levels.

Similarly, men with blood sugar levels in the upper 2.5 percent of normal fasting and two-hour glucose levels were approximately 1.8 times more likely to die from heart disease than men with low-normal blood glucose levels. This is *not* a coincidence.

SYMPTOMS OF A SILENT KILLER

The usual symptoms of a heart attack include a crushing feeling in the chest, pain in the chest (angina pectoris), pain radiating into the left arm and up into the jaw, and shortness of breath. However, it is also important to note that people with diabetes may not necessarily experience these symptoms all the time. Instead, symptoms that might occur include nausea, vomiting, tiredness, and sweating. Physicians call these symptoms "silent heart attacks." Silent heart attacks are more devastating than noticeable ones because lifesaving interventions might be delayed or might never be administered due to lack of detection.

The lesson here is that we shouldn't wait until a crisis pops up. Once you have metabolic syndrome, prediabetes, or diabetes, consult with your physician so that proper interventions may be instituted right away.

Heart attacks are not the only problem a severely diabetic person faces. Obesity also plays a role because it tends to overwork the heart and compromise its capacity to pump blood. Such complications may also be the result of high blood pressure and scarring caused by a heart attack. Among those with heart failure, 20 percent to 40 percent have diabetes.

ANOTHER LOOK AT BLOOD LIPIDS

Throughout this book, we have been tackling blood lipids: high-density lipoprotein (HDL) cholesterol, low-density lipoprotein (LDL) cholesterol, and triglycerides. It is good to review these diagnostic considerations to gain a better grasp of what to do in the case of abnormalities in these blood lipid levels, especially when talking about heart conditions.

Patients with metabolic syndrome, prediabetes, or Type 2 diabetes often have low HDL cholesterol, high triglyceride levels, or normal to heightened LDL cholesterol. Nevertheless, research has found that low HDL levels and high triglycerides are a recipe for a heart attack. If the goal is to lose weight, keep in mind that once you have problems with these lipids, controlling your intake of carbohydrate-rich food will be of major importance.

IS LDL CHOLESTEROL REALLY BAD FOR DIABETICS?

Having high levels of LDL cholesterol leads to a higher risk of vascular diseases due to clogged arteries, such as heart attack or stroke—hence the term *bad cholesterol*. Calling LDL cholesterol *bad* leads to simplicity, making it easier for pharmaceutical companies to sell drugs that limit cholesterol levels and prevent arteries from becoming blocked. When you take a closer look at LDL cholesterol, however, there is a more complicated mechanism at work.

The types of LDL cholesterol can be categorized as subfractions, depending on the size of the cholesterol particles. Very low-density lipoprotein particles are somewhat large, intermediate-density lipoproteins have smaller particles, and LDLs have the smallest particles of all. The smaller but denser molecules can be just as damaging to the arteries as other particles. For those with diabetes, metabolic syndrome, or prediabetes, the particles that are present are usually the smaller, denser LDL cholesterol, not the bigger, lighter, fluffier particles, which are less damaging. This is because high levels of insulin convert the production of cholesterol from the larger and lighter particles into the smaller, denser ones. Target your insulin levels by (1) consuming fewer carbohydrates, which will push your health in a positive direction, or by (2) loosening the particles of cholesterol already clogging your arteries.

For some diabetics, profuse LDL is comparatively modest and temporary, eventually becoming harmless. It can be periodically offset by improved HDL or triglyceride levels. The bottom line is that when you follow your doctor's guidelines, you can expect LDL to return to average levels in approximately three to six months. If your LDL rises again, ask your physician to lay out a plan. Prior to taking medications that can lower LDL cholesterol, why not ask your doctor how you got there in the first place?

Your physician might do a blood test for a certain lipid type known as lipoprotein, written as *lipoprotein(a)*, or *lp(a)* for short. This is another form of blood lipid known to be a risk factor for heart disease.

When your LDL cholesterol is satisfactory, your lp(a) levels could be elevated. Doctors believe the lp(a) level is inherited and cannot be altered through diet or other means. Nowadays, researchers are still looking into this facet of cardiac health to develop measures that could constrain the levels of this particular lipoprotein.

GOOD CHOLESTEROL: THE DIABETIC'S GUARDIAN

Opposite to LDL cholesterol is HDL cholesterol, also called the "good" or "protective" cholesterol. Known medically as high-density lipoprotein, this type of cholesterol is very active in clearing unused cholesterol from the bloodstream and carrying them to the liver. The higher the HDL level, the more cholesterol is filtered from the bloodstream before there is a chance of oxidation and damage to the blood vessels. This is why HDL cholesterol is the "good" cholesterol, not to mention that it protects the heart and arteries.

HDL particles come in various sizes, or subportions. Diabetics who have metabolic syndrome not only have lower levels of HDL, but their HDL type also tends to be in smaller and denser particles, more so than the LDL.

Also important are triglycerides and triacylglycerols, which are fat glob-ules that are present in almost all body fluids. High levels of these substances lead to undesirable effects in the body. According to Dr. Robert Atkins, the optimum number of triglycerides should be below one hundred. It is of great importance that carbohydrate intake be controlled; if it is not, your diet will consist mostly of triglycerides. When a diet consisting of low amounts of carbohydrates is adhered to consistently, you should see your general levels of triglycerides fall to a sensible number.

LDL CHOLESTEROL AND STATIN DRUGS

Because diabetic patients usually have average or only slightly elevated LDL levels, many will ask their doctor if they should strive to reduce their levels down to a low normal range. Some researchers say yes and believe that people with diabetes should be allowed to take statin drugs even if LDL is at standard levels.

Other physicians, such as Dr. Atkins, say no. They take it slowly since statin research has shown that a gradual reduction of LDL, even when it is not very high, can help people with diabetes to reduce their risk of heart disease. These studies do not prove that people need statin drugs to deal with both mild and serious cholesterol issues. After all, the research did not compare medications to diet control programs, which have a huge impact on improving a diabetic's lipid profile.

Diabetics experiencing heart complications may still benefit from drugs that fight high cholesterol and from following a rigid diet program. In doing so, you get a boost in the quality of your life as a diabetic.

REVISITING STATIN DRUGS

As mentioned earlier, statins are one popular classification of drugs for treating abnormal lipid levels. These are usually prescribed for people with metabolic syndrome, prediabetes, or diabetes. Patients with high cholesterol are typically prescribed these drugs because doctors are pressured to adhere to the National Cholesterol Education Program (NCEP), which dictates prescribing these medications. While many researchers have found them to be effective in removing cholesterol, there are advocates who prefer not to use these drugs for the prevention of heart disease and instead choose natural, holistic alternatives to medication.

In the past, statins were believed to lower cholesterol by blocking the manufacture of an enzyme that the body utilizes to make cholesterol. Due to recent research, however, some say that such effects may not really be connected to reducing cholesterol at all. Instead, statins work by limiting inflammation, especially of the epithelial cells that make up the lining of the blood vessels.

Whatever the true mechanisms of statin drugs, they must be monitored closely for any serious side effects. Statins halt the production of coenzyme Q_{10} (CoQ_{10}, or ubiquinone), a compound used in the metabolism of cells. Consuming too much of these drugs can result in damage to the liver and muscles, including the muscles of the heart. Damage to the muscles can turn out to be severe. The infamous drug Baychol was found to have caused multiple deaths, which led to its withdrawal from the market. Hepatic (liver) issues can result from the use of these drugs, so manufacturers suggest that blood tests be performed every three to six months in order to watch for evidence of liver damage.

Differences do not exist when comparing the use of statins for the purpose of keeping inflammation in check to the approach of targeting carbohydrates in the diet. Since high insulin levels contribute to inflammation, and since insulin levels are attributable to the levels of carbohydrates in the diet, the drug and diet approaches are equally effective.

Carbohydrate control can also help reduce excess inflammation in the body because secretions of homocysteine, an amino acid, contribute to the inflammation of cells along the blood vessel walls. People with low-carb diets also have reportedly low homocysteine levels. Likewise, helpful oils from the diet and supplements can also bring down inflammation, with or without the help of statins.

GOING FOR THE BLOOD LIPIDS

The third adult treatment panel of the NCEP provided new guidelines in 2001 for evaluating and treating high blood cholesterol. The panel issued a reduction of high cholesterol thresholds, adding many Americans to the list of those who need treatment with drugs—increasing the number from an estimated 15 million adults by the 1993 guidelines to around 36 million by the new guidelines. The panel also issued new low-fat, high-carbohydrate suggestions. These dietary recommendations cannot work without the patient losing weight, which means the patient will have to take more statin drugs.

The guidelines were derived from statistical data involving patients on a high–carbohydrate American diet. When blood glucose and insulin are over-abundant, the cells stop burning your lipids and begin storing the extra fat. By controlling carbohydrates, you prevent some of the hormonal effects of stored fat, resulting in high-risk complications to the cardiovascular system. This is why the Atkins diet is somewhat unhealthy despite being highly effective for weight loss.

In any case, here are the new NCEP guidelines:

LDL Cholesterol

Optimal	less than 100 mg/dL
Near optimal/above optimal	100–129 mg/dL
Borderline high	130–159 mg/dL
High	160–189 mg/dL
Very high	190 mg/dL or more

HDL Cholesterol

Low	less than 40 mg/dL
High	60 mg/dL or more

Total Cholesterol

Desirable	less than 200 mg/dL
Borderline high	200–239 mg/dL
High	240 mg/dL or more

Triglycerides

Normal	less than 150 mg/dL
Borderline high	150–199 mg/dL
High	200–499 mg/dL
Very high	500 mg/dL or more

ABDOMINAL FAT REVEALED

When treating diabetes and heart disease, cholesterol is like a very large parasite sitting on the diabetic's shoulder. Have you ever heard of anyone with healthy cholesterol readings suffering from a heart attack?

Note that heart attacks happen when blood flow to the arteries is blocked, most commonly by a major clot. Abdominal fat adds fuel to the fire by allowing for more chemicals that increase blood-clotting factors. This makes the platelets "stickier" and more likely to cause clotting.

If a diabetic has achieved satisfactory weight loss but still carries a lot of abdominal fat, they may be in for future heart troubles. Make sure you are disciplined in dealing with the situation and that you target the unused fat in your abdomen. The first goal is to make the HDL cholesterol counteractive against bad cholesterol. The second goal is to allow the general triglyceride levels to decrease. Clotting factors may also decrease since you have less fat.

Together with exercise routines, having the right amount of fat, lipids, and triglycerides in your bloodstream at all times will enable you to take charge of your diabetes.

OTHER RISK FACTORS FOR CHOLESTEROL

In addition to the factors already mentioned, try to observe the following three factors for improving your heart health as a diabetic.

Homocysteine

This is a typical by-product of the metabolism of methionine, an amino acid. If you have high levels of homocysteine in your blood, you risk getting heart disease from clogged arteries. At least 25 percent of the U.S. population is now at risk for death caused by some form of heart disease. This is genetic in nature. Having these genes puts you at a 2.5 times greater risk for heart disease.

Being a diabetic complicates matters. Even if you don't have the tendency in your genes to have high levels of homocysteine, with insulin resistance or diabetes, you will tend to have higher levels of this amino acid compared to those with normal glucose levels. You will also have a higher tendency for kidney disease.

C-reactive Protein

Inflammation creeps up on diabetics when there is an elevation in C-reactive protein (CRP) in the liver. As inflammation paves the way for the clotting of arteries, CRP increases are a warning that suggests heart disease.

In a study of males with high CRP levels, it was found that after about ten years these men suffered more heart attacks compared to those who had normal levels of CRP. Identical results were found in the Nurses' Health Study mentioned earlier.

Type 2 diabetics with abdominal fat and impaired glucose tolerance usually end up with high CRP levels. Acute illness or hormone therapy can also lead to high CRP levels.

Worried? Don't be. According to research involving overweight women with high levels of inflammation, patients who lost around 10 percent of their body weight from exercise and nutrition therapy reported a substantial decrease in their CRP levels, leading to a healthier heart. In fact, the CRP in these individuals decreased to levels similar to those of patients with acceptable body weight.

Fibrinogen

Fibrinogen is a blood protein that partially accounts for the process of blood clotting. When levels of fibrinogen are high, the blood may clot very easily. Such clotting may lead to arterial blockage, heart attack, and other related illnesses. Those with diabetes, prediabetes, and metabolic syndrome all have elevated levels of fibrinogen, a statistic that is similar to that of other chemicals involved in blood clotting. This inclination toward blood clotting may also be connected with abnormal inflammatory processes that are part of metabolic syndrome. Increased fibrinogen levels interact with other factors such as birth control medications and hormonal imbalances. This is primarily why many doctors prescribe low-dose aspirin, highly regarded as an all-in-one fix, to reduce the risk of heart disease caused by high fibrinogen levels.

MEDICATIONS THAT LOWER HEART ATTACK RISK

Reducing the causes of heart disease and stroke as soon as possible is vital. This leads us to three goals:

- Tackle the bad cholesterol levels and raise the good ones.
- Decrease blood pressure, which is often high in those at risk for diabetes.
- Reduce the risk for blood clotting and the formation of harmful plaques in the arteries.

Also consider different medications and other alternatives to help reduce these potential risks according to the recommendations of your doctor.

If you recall, we have already discussed statins. Some examples are pravastatin (Pravachol), simvastatin (Zocor), fluvastatin (Lescol), lovastatin (Mevacor), atorvastatin (Lipitor), rosuvastatin (Crestor), and Ezetimibe (Zetia).

Drugs that modify triglyceride levels include niacin (Niaspan) and fibric acid derivatives like gemfibrozil (Lopid).

To reduce your problems with high blood pressure, there are angiotensin converting enzyme (ACE) inhibitors such as benazepril (Lotensin), lisinopril (Zestril), ramipril (Altace), and enalapril (Vasotec), which do a fairly good job.

Aspirin and clopidogrel (Plavix) also help reduce the risk of blood clotting. Aspirin should be taken in low doses first to make sure the body does not get overwhelmed with any possible side effect. Physicians suggest around eighty-one milligrams a day. You also have the choice of taking an enteric-coated form of aspirin which is more easygoing for the stomach.

Experts say that the chance of having a heart attack or stroke is reduced by 30 percent if the patient takes the advisable amount of aspirin daily. For patients at high risk for having a heart attack and other related issues, the dose is elevated to the 325 milligrams of an adult-strength tablet per day.

The difficulty with aspirin is that it causes a predisposition for bruising and bleeding. It is also very rough on the stomach and can lead to ulcers and other gastrointestinal troubles. These issues, however, occur infrequently and are outweighed by the benefits.

With respect to drugs that decrease triglyceride levels, such as Lopid and Tricor, remember that using these drugs can reduce one's vulnerability for having a heart attack. Even if statins are prescribed more often than Lopid and Tricor, these drugs have many benefits, including fewer side effects. For example, they don't cause occasional muscle pain like statins do. However, like statins, they may result in liver problems. If these drugs are to be used in combination with statins, Tricor is preferable over Lopid, since it is less likely to have effects on the muscles.

Two other drugs are important for the treatment of metabolic syndrome: angiotensin converting enzyme (ACE) inhibitors and angiotensin receptor blockers (ARBs). ACE inhibitors limit the action of the enzyme that converts angiotensin, a hormone related to hypertension, into an active form called renin. Lower blood pressure results, and the blood vessels become less irritated and inflamed.

Physicians know that ACE inhibitors and ARBs work by reversing the high level of inflammation in the blood vessels. This inflammation leads to a higher risk of clots and thus heart attacks. ACE inhibitors also tend to have positive effects on the kidneys.

Just like any other blood pressure drug, ACE inhibitors do have side effects, including an annoying dry cough. When this occurs, patients can switch to a drug classified as an ARB, which does not cause coughing as a major side effect.

Another side effect of ACE inhibitors is hyperkalemia, which is an elevation in potassium levels. This is alarming when it occurs, so you have to have your blood tested four to six weeks after starting on this drug.

Angiotensin receptor blockers (ARBs) are the last of the drugs employed against metabolic syndrome. They function just like ACE inhibitors, and though they don't cause coughing as a side effect, they do result in increased overall potassium levels.

REVIEWING THE MACROVASCULAR COMPLICATIONS

As noted earlier, the heart's relation to diabetes takes the form of macrovascular complications. There are changes that take place in the medium and large blood vessels. The blood vessels thicken, sclerose (harden), and become blocked by plaque that sticks to the walls of the vessels. Thus blood flow can be severely reduced.

Studies are still being done to complete our understanding of the connection between hyperglycemia and atherosclerosis. Other factors are known to be linked with atherosclerosis, such as obesity, high levels of triglycerides, and high blood pressure. You can manage these factors with healthy diet and exercise. Hypertension and hyperlipidemia can also be avoided in this manner.

SUPPLEMENTS FOR CARDIAC HEALTH

Besides medications for preventing the occurrence of heart disease, various supplements can also be taken to help diabetic patients. For those with a high risk of heart disease, prediabetes, diabetes, and metabolic syndrome, doctors recommend taking different supplements that serve as antioxidants and boost health.

Vitamin C

With high levels of vitamin C, the blood vessels tend to relax, allowing blood to flow through smoothly. If you have high levels of blood sugar together with high blood pressure, they can be kept under control by taking vitamin C. The dosage varies from one thousand to two thousand milligrams per day.

Vitamin E

Diabetics with severe sugar abnormalities can benefit greatly from vitamin E supplements, since they help prevent LDL cholesterol from oxidizing too many radicals. Vitamin E also helps decrease the risk of clogged arteries. It makes the blood less sticky, which helps prevent the occurrence of heart attack–inducing blood clots.

B Vitamins

You really need three B vitamins for a fit heart and sustainable blood sugar. First is folic acid, sometimes referred to as folate.

Second, supplements abundant in folic acid together with vitamin B_{12} (cobalamin) lead to favorable levels of homocysteine by helping out the enzymes that break down sugars.

Vitamin B_3 is also beneficial. This supplement is now improved because of the development of a form of this vitamin known as inositol hexanicotinate (IHN). This works well without the unpleasant side effects of large doses of niacin. However, niacin and IHN cause an elevation of glucose levels if you have diabetes.

Panthenine, another form of B vitamin, also known as pantothenic acid, may also be helpful for controlling total cholesterol and LDL, and it has minimal side effects.

Magnesium

If you have metabolic syndrome, prediabetes, or diabetes, your levels of magnesium can become very low. Besides being bad for your diabetes, this is bad for your blood pressure and your heart. Low levels of magnesium can result in heart arrhythmias, or irregular heartbeat, also making your blood stickier and prone to clot formation. Magnesium can also affect blood pressure.

Hypomagnesemia, in which the walls of the blood vessels become tightened, leads to an increase in blood pressure. Magnesium helps keep the blood vessels relaxed, thus reducing blood pressure. If you have kidney disease, it will also be helpful if you take magnesium supplements as advised by your physician.

Taurine

Taurine, an amino acid, is also vital for treating high blood pressure because it acts as a natural diuretic, leading you to excrete fluid. Blood pressure then goes down, and there is less strain on the heart. Taurine also enhances immunity, as it protects against oxidative stress. It usually comes in 500 milligram tablets, and the dose range is usually from 1,500 to 3,000 milligrams per day, divided into three doses.

Essential Fatty Acids

Omega-3 fatty acids play a fundamental role in avoiding heart disease for diabetes because they function to decrease the levels of triglycerides and reduce blood pressure. Foods with a high content of these fatty acids include fish, which you should eat at least twice a week.

It is also known that omega-3 is good for countering high blood pressure. If you want to receive all of the omega-3 fatty acids, like eicosapentaenoic acid (EPA) and docosahexaenoic acid (DHA), which are found only in fish oil, then take a soft gel with six hundred milligrams of fish oil. The dosage can then be modified to two or four soft gels a day. If triglyceride levels are really high, there is need for higher doses until the lab's results indicate an optimum level of triglycerides. If you are planning to take medications to thin your blood, you should ask your physician first. The idea is to try to balance your intake of omega-3 and omega-6 fatty acids (also known as gamma linolenic acid, or GLA).

Coenzyme Q_{10}

A negative side-effect of taking statin drugs (those taken to reverse high cholesterol levels) is their interference with the production of coenzyme Q_{10} (ubiquinone, or CoQ_{10}). Since you need this coenzyme to be able to make energy in the mitochondria, the "power plant" of the cell, there could be fatigue and muscle weakness if this molecule falls short of the required levels. This is just a minor repercussion. As a major effect, note that a decline in coenzyme Q_{10} will lead to difficulties with your heart, as the heart contains more of this coenzyme than any other part of the body.

GETTING YOUR HEART FIT

Just like you perform exercise routines to keep your muscles healthy, you can do much better with your health if you learn how to sustain a healthy disposition and fitness through various exercises involving different parts of the body. This is what a holistic approach is about. You can treat your cardiovascular system like a king through discipline and knowledge of the proper means to deal with heart disease.

Aerobic exercise boosts stamina and fitness levels while providing energy and extending the lifespan. In your daily life, you will always have need for extra heart and lung capacity. Although colds, the flu, and even bronchitis and pneumonia may occur, they will only be an inconvenience since your metabolism will be efficient and will allow your body to repel the symptoms of any affliction.

You can get optimal physical results by doing cardiovascular workouts for sixty minutes each day. When your body gets used to such workouts, the exercise can be more vigorous depending on your body's capacity. It is best to do weight-bearing exercises, like brisk walking (at a minimum of four miles per hour), cross-country skiing, jogging, rollerblading, snow shoeing, or playing basketball, soccer, racquetball, or squash. If you can maintain a steady pace, you may also chop wood or carry water. You can also work in the garden by raking, hoeing, and weeding.

Strict, routine exercise matters (for around fifteen to twenty minutes), as burning fat and energy is one of the healthiest things you can do as a diabetes patient with heart disease. Walking to and from the corners of a parking lot, running up and down the stairs of your office, and riding your bicycle all serve as great additions to your everyday workout.

Find an activity you can stick to and that you enjoy. Make this activity a priority, just like eating and sleeping are essential components of daily life. Are you willing to devote time to improve your health and to endure sacrifice that really counts?

Join a sports league that will suit your interest and develop your health. Also make sure the activity you are planning to do is in line with your capability, age, and other factors. If you are forty or older, it would be safer to undergo a stress test to determine the level of exercise your heart can take before embarking on an exercise routine. This is also advised if you have a family history of cardiac disease.

Maximum Heart Rate

To determine the maximum recommended heart rate for exercising, just subtract your age from 220 beats per minute (bpm). If you are forty years old, the highest recommended heart rate is 220 bpm minus 40, or 180 bpm.

Shoot for 70 percent to 85 percent of the highest rate as your goal. Maintain that rate for about twenty minutes per session. If you are forty, determine your highest and lowest attainable heart rates for exercising by taking 70 percent of 180 bpm, which is 126 bpm, and 85 percent of 180 bpm, which would be 153 bpm. Based on these calculations, you will want to exercise at 126 to 153 bpm for around twenty minutes. If you are able to do this a minimum of three times every week, you will soon achieve the benefits of proper discipline.

The good thing about targeting your heart rate is that it automatically reveals your level of fitness. As you get increasingly fit, you will have to do more rigorous exercises to be able to achieve your target heart rate, thereby helping you to reach your fitness goals. This will subsequently encourage you to be more active and to discover your true physical potential as a diabetic with heart disease.

Part Four

DEALING WITH DIABETES

• 9 •

The Diabetic's Ultimate Diet

$\mathcal{D}$iabetes and diet go together like peanut butter and jelly. In case you are wondering why we've been talking about carbohydrates and other nutrients, and about foods that can combat diabetes as well as those that can trigger the occurrence of this illness, it is because this allows us to handle such a silent killer with more confidence.

For years, carbohydrates have been seen as an enemy of diabetes patients. The influence of carbohydrates on glucose has been discussed in previous chapters, but one must also take into account the amount of carbohydrates that are consumed from a practical standpoint. Additional information must be considered when trying to determine the best diet out there for diabetics.

GIVING DIET THERAPY A SHOT

In Type 2 diabetes, the main purpose of diet therapy is to restore optimum insulin functioning by counteracting insulin resistance. Changes in your diet and lifestyle will help you achieve this goal, by losing weight and increasing physical activity. There are three primary goals:

- To protect against heart disease
- To develop healthy body weight
- To achieve and maintain ideal blood glucose levels

The purpose of these goals is to decrease the incidence of short- and long-term complications connected with diabetes. These complications include diseases

143

that affect the eyes, kidneys, nerves, heart, and blood vessels. Thus these goals help a person to improve the quality of their life and general health.

In light of this, let's identify the different diets necessary for preventing the various conditions that may arise in diabetes.

GOAL 1: PROTECTION FROM HEART DISEASE

Your condition as a diabetic is top priority, so careful consideration of your food intake will forever be in your best interest. This is how you can keep your organs active and healthy. The most notable recommendation for a healthy diet is the American Heart Association's "heart healthy" or "prudent" diet. You get less than 30 percent of calories from fat, 10 percent of calories from saturated fat, and three hundred milligrams of total cholesterol. However, even though this diet has been known for reducing the incidence of heart disease, its effectiveness in the treatment of diabetes is unimpressive. This is why, by and large, you will experience better results with the very low-fat vegetarian diets and the relatively low-fat Mediterranean diets.

Very Low-Fat Vegetarian Diets

The low-fat vegetarian and vegan diets have both been proven to be strong in the battle against heart disease. Countless researchers have worked to discover that not only do these diets curb the levels of cholesterol, but they also reverse the usual course of high cholesterol.

This sort of diet contains a variety of vegetables, fruits, legumes, and whole grains. Additional fats of any type, such as oils, margarine, shortening, mayonnaise, and oil-based salad dressings, are almost completely avoided. Plant foods with higher fat content, such as seeds, avocados, nuts, and olives are restricted if not completely eliminated. The total fat content should not exceed 10 percent of the calories, with saturated fat at about 2 percent. Some of the very low-fat diets like this include tiny amounts of egg whites and non-fat milk products. Meanwhile, other programs are very strict when it comes to the vegan diet, with no consumption of eggs, dairy products, or meat.

Low-Fat, Mediterranean-Style Diets

Diet-savvy patients wonder how high-fat diets can be very effective at controlling the level of blood sugar since these diets also tend to be low in carbohydrates. Owing to their high content of good fat and low amounts of bad fat, Mediterranean-style diets lead us to think that they will actually cause damage to the heart, but this is not always the case. According to medical research, not all high-fat diets cause heart damage. Some such diets may actually take the heart under its wing and protect it. So, what does the Mediterranean diet *really* involve?

Considering the details of this diet, we might notice that it focuses on a certain assortment of foods. These foods usually undergo minimal commercial processing, and if possible are seasonally fresh and grown locally. As a daily dessert, fresh fruits are usually the choice, with sweets eaten only a few times a week. Hey, a few times is better than none! Olive oil serves as the main source of fat, and shortening, margarine, butter, and other forms of hard fat are not used much. The total fat consumed should be around 30 to 35 percent of calories, and not in excess of 7 to 8 percent saturated fat.

Food items from animals are supposed to be eaten in moderation, and red meat should be consumed only a few times a month. There is slightly more poultry involved in these diets than red meat, while fish is eaten two to three times a week. No more than four eggs should be consumed per week. Even if it is okay for you to eat dairy, your dairy diet should principally be cheese and yogurt. Alcohol should be limited as much as possible. It should normally be consumed with meals, and should be around one to two glasses a day for men and a glass a day for women.

The Sense of These Two Diets

Why are Mediterranean and very low-fat vegetarian diets recommended as healthy for heart disease and diabetes patients? They are, in fact, very different from the majority of diets found today.

To begin, although the Mediterranean-style and the very low-fat vegetarian diets have different amounts of total fat, they are actually comprised of the same food content. This is true especially because both diets are based on legumes, vegetables, whole grains, and fruits. The two diets also provide plenty of plant protein, vitamins, fiber, minerals, and other compounds necessary for a healthy body and a healthy heart. It's a sure thing that they are also both low in bad fat, with no saturated trans fat or cholesterol, which are all agents of disease. Their main difference involves the use of olive oil in the Mediterranean program, while in the very low-fat vegetarian diet, higher-fat plant foods like nuts, seeds, olives, and avocados are considered. Even if these are consumed, they still promote good cardiac health.

Very Low-Fat Diets: When Getting Skinny Doesn't Cut It

If you think about very low-fat diets in relation to Type 2 diabetes, you will likely encounter four issues. First, these diets may not provide an adequate amount of long-chain omega-3 fatty acids, which are usually found in fish oil, walnuts, flax seeds, and green leafy vegetables. These omega-3 fatty acids have been shown to provide needed protection from heart disease. They decrease the levels of triglycerides and reduce the risk of blood clotting, and they prevent the occurrence of irregular heartbeats. The protective capabilities of specific molecules mean a lot when it comes to diabetes. If there are insufficient quantities of these molecules, there will be a higher risk of heart disease. Very low-fat vegetarian diets lack fat except what is found in foods like soy products, seeds, and nuts. These foods only provide around 25 to 30 percent of the omega-3 fatty acids an individual needs.

Second, keep in mind the absorption of fat-soluble vitamins, minerals, and phytochemicals (phytochemicals are the strong, healthy chemicals found in plants). Research studies have shown that the absorption of particular nutrients is enhanced by a moderate intake of fat in the diet. Fat-soluble vitamins like vitamin E, substances known as carotenoids (vitamin A), some minerals, and phytochemicals help with absorption of other nutrients. These dietary constituents are very important for people suffering from diabetes and should therefore be included in any diet.

Third, note the considerable reduction in the nutritional content of the food. If you tend to pick through nutrition facts labels, this is very important! Diabetics who severely restrict their fat intake lose the richest sources of vitamin E, other trace minerals, protective phytochemicals, and selenium, which is plentiful in foods like seeds, nuts, avocados, olives, and even fat-brimming soy products.

Fourth, remember that diets with very low-fat and highly refined carbohydrates can lead to very low levels of HDL cholesterol, as well as notable increases in triglycerides. When this occurs in conjunction with diabetes, there is a high risk for heart disease. These problems are caused by carbohydrates found in various refined foods, such as white flour products and foods high in sugar. With whole grains in your diet, the changes in HDL and triglycerides can be minimized. According to various studies, whole food diets that are high in carbohydrates reduce triglyceride levels. Such diets may have varying effects on HDL cholesterol levels.

The Problem with High-Fat Diets

You might run into some of the following complications with high-fat diets in combination with Type 2 diabetes:

- High-fat diets are linked to insulin resistance and the production of weak insulin. Diets with saturated fat are the most problematic in this area. With regard to insulin secretion, trans-fatty acids cause the most trouble.

- High-fat diets can lead to obesity. When fats are constantly ingested, they can eventually add up to more than twice the calories contained in proteins or carbohydrates. Since fat has less bulk, a person may have a tendency to eat and eat until they are too full. Likewise, dietary fat may also be stored as body fat, something that is not as easily done with carbohydrates or protein. The number of obesity cases grows when these fats are so close at hand. Don't forget that there is also a higher risk for just about any chronic disease with high-fat diets.
- High-fat diets can result in dilution of nutrient density, making it difficult to meet standard nutrient recommendations. This becomes a concern for people who are watching their weight and would like to keep their calories within certain bounds. This dilemma is made more complicated because the primary sources of fat are concentrated in vegetable oils, margarine, butter, and mayonnaise. Foods without added fats (like nuts, seeds, soy, avocados, and other whole foods) stay on the healthy side. Fats and oils that are refined through intense manufacturing processes contain virtually no vitamins, protein, minerals, fiber, or other protective substances like vitamin E. When consumed in large amounts, high-fat foods make it difficult to meet the nutritional needs of the body due to interference with nutrients that are already scarce, such as calcium and magnesium.
- High-fat diets may lead to serious oxidative damage to the body's tissues. To counteract this, we need to get rid of the free radicals circulating around in our system. Free radicals are highly energized oxygen molecules carrying one or more unpaired electrons. When these electrons react abruptly with other molecules, they turn into free radicals, resulting in a destructive chain of events that causes oxidative damage to the body's tissues. Free radicals react with dangerously unstable substances when you consume large amounts of fat and only a small amount of antioxidants from plant foods. Simply put, there is a greater chance that oxidative damage will occur as a result of high-fat diets. When this form of oxidative stress takes place, various diseases become more likely, such as heart disease, cancer, diabetes, arthritis, and neurological disorders.

GOAL 2: PROMOTION OF HEALTHY WEIGHT

The second aim of a diabetic diet is the maintenance of a healthy and desirable weight. This is because 80 percent of people with Type 2 diabetes are overweight, and 40 percent are obese.

You may not realize it, but insulin resistance is triggered as fat accumulates in the body. Being overweight can lead to high blood pressure and heart disease. According to various research studies, weight loss in people with Type 2 diabetes reduces insulin resistance associated with decreased blood sugar. The loss of pounds also seems to reduce blood cholesterol and triglyceride levels, as well as systolic and diastolic blood pressure. You might want to set a specific goal for how much weight you want to lose in diet therapy. There is nothing like the sense of accomplishment a diabetic gets when he or she loses the desired amount of weight. In addition to diabetes, weight loss works very well against several other diseases.

What types of diets are perfect for such goals? For starters, you can use whole foods, high fiber, and plant-based nutrients in your diet. For obvious reasons, high fat intake is related to the body's "fatness." Studies suggest that, even with unrestricted consumption of low-fat and unprocessed plant foods like fruits, vegetables, whole grains, and beans, there are still possibilities for major weight loss. There is plenty of hope for those who want to lose weight after all.

A moderately low-fat diet is recommended if you get around 20 to 25 percent of your calories from fat. For example, a 2,200-calorie diet provides fifty to sixty-five grams of fat per day. This puts you almost halfway between the Mediterranean-style diet and the very low-fat vegetarian diet. To make full use of essential fatty acids, mineral absorption, and total nutritional quality, plant foods with higher fat contents, like nuts, seeds, olives, and avocados, should be limited as much as possible. There may be small amounts of high-quality oils like extra virgin olive oil. If we look more closely at the regimen for weight loss, diet is only half of the struggle against diabetes. Exercise should also be taken into consideration.

GOAL 3: CONTROL OF BLOOD SUGAR

The third and final goal pertains to the control of blood sugar levels. If not controlled well, there can be complications for the eyes, kidneys, nerves, and other parts of the body. To promote healthy control of blood glucose levels, we can start by knowing about the food items that influence sugar levels the most. Observe how much your sugar levels go up from eating certain foods, and observe how fast they go up. You also need to know the dynamics of nondietary approaches like exercise and stress management. Certain factors related to diet may have considerable effects on blood sugar, including carbohydrates, fiber, fats, and the frequency of eating.

CARBOHYDRATES AND DIABETES

Though we discussed carbohydrates earlier on, we will deal with them further in this chapter because they really are one of the stars in the topic of diet therapy.

Carbohydrates have the most impact on the levels of sugar in the blood. With no surprise, we know that carbohydrates are different forms of the same basic molecule known as sugar. Many diabetics today think that simple sugars or simple carbohydrates are the bad ones while complex sugars or complex carbohydrates cause less damage. If we really analyze the facts, though, this is plainly inaccurate. Read on to find out why this is so!

Simple carbohydrates can be found in refined, nutrient-depleted foods, but they can also be found in nutrient-rich whole foods like fruits and vegetables. Meanwhile, complex carbohydrates can be found in heavily processed foods like wheat bread and pastries, but they can also be found in nutrient-dense foods like wheat berries and beans. Our glycemic (sugar) reaction to carbohydrates depends on several factors, including the following:

- *The number of grams of carbohydrates available.* The denser the carbohydrates, the higher the blood sugar level will be.
- *The type of sugar (glucose, sucrose, fructose, lactose).* Glucose leads to an elevated glycemic index compared to sucrose (table sugar), lactose (milk sugar), or fructose (fruit sugar).
- *The type of starch (amylose or amylopectin).* Indeed, various types of starch are present in the different food items consumed from day to day. Amylopectin has the capacity to be absorbed and broken down, in contrast to amylose. Starchy foods differ in their starch content and characteristics. For instance, rice has more amylopectin than pasta, and thus it has greater tendencies to cause blood sugar to rise.
- *The amount of fiber.* Diets high in fiber can slow down the absorption of carbohydrates. Insoluble fiber slows the process down more than soluble fiber does.
- *The type of preparation (cooked, raw, liquid, dry, paste, ground, or otherwise processed).* Processing and cooking can change the sugar content of foods drastically. Cooking makes the sugar molecules less dense and can thereby moderate the effects on the blood sugar of diabetics. High-density foods cannot increase a person's carbohydrates as easily in comparison to low-density products. Thus pasta would cause a smaller increase in glucose than bread.
- *The presence of other nutrients in certain foods.* Fat and other components of food have the capacity to slow digestion. Chocolate, which is rich

in both fat and sugar, can at times be better on blood sugar than brown rice. However, most patients believe that eating brown rice is more advisable than consuming huge amounts of chocolate.

The glycemic index (GI) provides the information needed for understanding the direct effects of food on blood sugar. This is a means of categorizing foods depending on their ability to control severe diabetes, broadly speaking.

Test meals are fed to the patient in portions containing fifty grams of carbohydrates. Blood sugar levels are carefully measured for three hours after ingesting the sample food. A response curve is plotted. This graph shows the sugar levels reached and the length of time they remained at those levels. This result is then compared to a standard reference curve of another food, which in most cases is glucose or white bread. The standard food is given a value of one hundred, while the test food value is given as a comparative percentage for how high and for how long the test food increased blood sugar levels.

Note that the GI does not simply measure the length of time the sugar remains in the bloodstream or how high the peak of the curve becomes. The more glucose that enters the blood in the first three hours, the higher the GI will be.

The GI is far from perfect, all things considered. It should be used together with other factors, like total nutritional value and food content.

Another measurement, known as glycemic load (GL), is thought to be the new measure of choice. It is defined as the amount of carbohydrates present in a food multiplied by the GI. Thus it gives a more meaningful measure of the glycemic burden of food by considering the amount of carbohydrates taken in. The GL of a small amount of food with a high GI can be as great as a larger amount of food with a lower GI. Get it? While GL is not as well known or commonly used, diets with a high GL are believed to increase the risk of developing Type 2 diabetes. Such diets also tend to increase HDL cholesterol levels.

FIBER IS NOTHING TO FEAR

For a very long time, researchers have debated the effect of fiber on blood sugar. It is known that fiber has a slowing effect on the absorption of carbohydrates and blood glucose. The effects of fiber are actually considered moderate unless consumption is higher than normal. Still, the positive effects are provided via soluble fiber. Research indicates the following:

- Ten to twenty grams of fiber per day has a minor impact on glycemic (sugar) control. This is the usual amount consumed by the average North American.
- Twenty to thirty-five grams of fiber per day leads to better glycemic control. For serious diets, ten to twenty more grams of fiber should be consumed. This is the amount suggested for good health in general, not just for diabetics.
- Thirty-five to fifty grams of fiber per day has excellent effects on glycemic control. Lacto-ovo vegetarians consume around thirty to forty grams of fiber every day, and vegans consume around forty to fifty grams a day.

Lacto-ovo vegetarians are those who do not eat meat, fish, or poultry but do eat dairy products and eggs. Vegans, with some similarities, have a few differences. Vegans prefer not to eat anything from animals. Eggs, dairy products, gelatin (made from the bones and connective tissues of animals), and the sweet honey we all long for are likely to be out of the question.

Fiber is a form of carbohydrate that is considered to be largely undigestible, meaning that it cannot be broken down and converted to blood glucose with ease. Fiber clogs up the digestive processes in the intestines. Research has shown that it also decreases levels of glucose and permits the transfer of fat to the blood after eating, but excessive fiber in the diet can be damaging for a diabetes patient.

Fiber, when consumed in the right amounts, can have some really good effects on your metabolism and digestive system. The more fiber there is, the lower the GI will be in the food one eats, since fiber itself reduces blood sugar levels. If whatever you are eating is not too processed and overflowing with preservatives, the fiber you eat will eventually be metabolized. Fiber counteracts the metabolism processes of the food we usually eat, so it allows more food to be absorbed by the bowels.

Americans unfortunately do not get enough fiber in their diets. Adults should consume around twenty to thirty-five grams of fiber a day. Having more fiber in the diet helps you lose weight, and you also lose cholesterol in the process. When you increase your daily consumption of fiber, be sure to drink adequate amounts of fluid to prevent the dreadful feeling of constipation.

Various sources of soluble fiber can be found in oats and oatmeal, oat bran, corn and rice bran, barley, dried beans, kidney beans, black beans, and pinto beans. On the other hand, insoluble fiber can be found in whole grains and whole-grain products (such as pasta, cereal, bread, and crackers), as well as in fresh fruit, vegetables, and brown rice.

FATS

Fats do not require any insulin to be metabolized, but can we really say that high-fat diets are good for glycemic control? When we look closely at fats, we see that there are more details in how fat is used than meet the eye. We also have to consider the amount and type of fat, both of which may interact with glucose tolerance and insulin sensitivity.

Amount of Fat

High-fat diets can result in reduced glucose tolerance by impairing the ability of insulin to bind with insulin receptors, which leads to insulin resistance. There may also be reduced sugar transport through the cells. Studies have shown that high-fat foods are noticeably associated with insulin resistance, whereas whole foods and high-carb diets are not.

Type of Fat

Digging deeper into diabetes, diet, and heart disease risk factors, there should be no doubt that the type of fat is just as important as the amount. Specifically, we are focusing on the fat present in our tissues, which may also push fluids out through the cell membranes and impair the functioning of insulin.

- Saturated fat—Intake of saturated fat is associated with a greater risk of glucose intolerance and increased fasting glucose and insulin levels. Likewise, elevated amounts of saturated fats in the body have been linked to higher levels of insulin and weakened sensitivity to insulin, and hence a greater risk of developing Type 2 diabetes.
- Unsaturated fat—Diets abundant in monounsaturated and polyunsaturated fats like olive oil and other vegetable oils are linked to a lower risk of Type 2 diabetes and lower fasting blood sugar levels. Higher levels of long-chain polyunsaturated fats in particular body tissues are linked with better insulin sensitivity. Thus, replacing saturated with monounsaturated fat is one option for promoting better insulin sensitivity. For those with high-fat diets, the beneficial effects of this type of fat type may be lost.
- Trans-fatty acids—Research studies on the effects of this type of fat are limited. Amidst all the scientific evidence that trans-fatty acids result in a significant increase in insulin secretion, there is still no hard evidence with regard to glycemic control. There is reason to believe this type of fat leads to a higher risk of Type 2 diabetes and heart disease.

With this knowledge, let's choose wisely the food we consume, and as we learn about the effects of fat on diabetes, let us think about what it does for a diabetic's overall health.

EATING FREQUENCY

What about the complication that people generally do not eat the same amount of food each day? Does that really matter? If you snack often, will it be good for your diabetes situation or will it be harmful?

Decades of research suggest that increasing the frequency of smaller meals leads to proper limitation of blood sugar, especially for those with Type 1 diabetes. It is better for diabetics with Type 1 to eat more frequently during the course of the day. Recent research has also shown that eating more often in smaller quantities is beneficial for Type 2 diabetics as well.

On a positive note, it has been discovered that when comparing "nibbling" diets with diets of three large meals and a snack, the nibbling diet proves to be healthier from a diabetic's point of view. It encourages improved glycemic control compared to the so-called healthy diet. Another study was carried out in which researchers found that with six tiny meals a day, changes in blood sugar were less common, and blood sugar was less likely to peak.

On the negative side, these studies did not show further positive effects of small but frequent meals. Differences between three-meal and nine-meal regimens were observed for four weeks, but these studies did not look at differences in glycemic control or insulin response. There were no significant differences in overall levels of blood glucose or the secretion of insulin.

Diabetics wonder how often they should eat. Should they have two colossal meals a day or five smaller ones? Increasing the frequency of meals from three to around five or six meals a day can help moderate the extremes of blood sugars and will help control the insulin response.

So, are there any noteworthy conclusions we can draw from this?

Yes. Increasing your meals does help you regulate your blood sugar, provided the change does not result in out-of-control weight gain. Therefore, since an increase in weight can lead to serious concerns for those with Type 2 diabetes, moderation should be practiced.

COUNTING CARBOHYDRATES IN TYPE 1 DIABETES

Learning to count carbohydrates is a good habit to follow if you want to counteract Type 1 diabetes. Once you incorporate this habit into your life, you might feel better by simply knowing you are eating the right amount of nutrients.

It may take months or even years to get used to monitoring your carbohydrate intake so that you can cope more successfully with diabetes. You will have to make use of various strategies that will help you carry out proper dieting. Besides books containing information on carbohydrate monitoring, you can use instruments called food-measuring scales. These scales are like guides to use when calculating your food. They provide a visual representation of what fifteen grams of rice or pasta really looks like. You can also use measuring cups, since they let you specify how much of a particular food you are taking in.

Once you have the necessary tools, you can prepare meals based on how many grams of carbohydrates are present in various foods. You can also precalculate your insulin dose to match the carbohydrates you are consuming. Over time, you may end up memorizing the amount of carbohydrates in the foods you eat.

Did you know that the tip of your thumb is about a teaspoonful, and you can use it to measure the ounces of almost any substance? Palms differ a lot more in size than fingertips, and while a man's palm can hold three to four servings, a woman's fist is more like two or three. This is equivalent to one to two cups of liquid volume.

To summarize, there is a wide assortment of carbohydrate monitoring options you can take advantage of without depleting your savings account. Remember that such tools are always available as long as you are willing to learn about them and apply them in your everyday life.

THE BIG IDEA ABOUT CARBOHYDRATES

We have been talking about carbohydrates since the beginning of this chapter. We talked about how to reduce carbohydrates for a better life. However, we need to take a closer look at carbohydrates to get a better idea of the exact food items we can or cannot eat. This also allows you to be more prepared for what is in store for you if you are a newly diagnosed diabetic.

In the long struggle against diabetes, eating homemade meals and avoiding restaurants is very important. Otherwise you will be largely unaware of what you are consuming. The goal is to take control of the carbohydrates in your diet at all times.

Preparing Starches

Measuring the amount of starch in your diet is very important, so you should master the art of measuring portion sizes. In basic terms, the ideal cooking size is around half a cup of cooked starch. To see what this looks like, measure half a cup of pasta or potatoes. Half-cup servings are typically equivalent to fifteen grams of carbohydrates, except for rice. Because uncooked rice is dense in its natural form, one third of a cup of rice is equal to about fifteen grams of carbohydrates.

Other servings equivalent to fifteen grams of carbohydrates include one slice of bread or half a cup of potatoes, kidney beans, garbanzo beans, lima beans, squash, peas, croutons, lentils, or corn. Many starches are mingled into salads or cooked with other dishes, so it is good to gauge fifteen grams at home to have an idea of what it looks like when it is served with restaurant food.

The Fruit Connection

We learned before that fruits are also good sources of carbohydrates because they are filled with different nutrients, vitamins, and minerals. Even if fruit sugar can lead to high levels of blood sugar, fresh fruit contains adequate fiber to suppress the elevation. Thus when fruit is cooked or mashed, like when you make your favorite fruit juice, your overall carbohydrates spike and then decrease quickly. Dietary fiber, on the other hand, will diminish slowly.

Eat fresh fruits whenever you can, with the exception of fruits like bananas. Bananas can increase your blood sugar to unwanted levels. In fact, if you measure the carbohydrate content of a banana, you might be surprised to find out that the recommended allowance of carbohydrates can be satisfied by eating only half a banana. An entire banana has about two servings, or thirty grams, of carbohydrates.

An obstacle you need to overcome when measuring fruit carbohydrates is that the natural sizes of fruits are obviously not premeasured. Even if the fruits in the grocery store seem similar in size, natural fruits always vary in carbohydrate content. Owing to the different stages of ripening found in nature, sweetness is not an observable characteristic of fruit. Regardless of the actual size, experts recommend daily consumption of around two to four servings of fruit per day.

You are probably wondering how to add fruits to your diet when there are so many gourmet options on the menu. Simply remember, a very small apple, a small peach, or a small pear is equal to fifteen grams of carbohydrates. If you find large ones at the store, you may have to count them as twenty or twenty-five grams of carbohydrates. Eating a whole banana or grapefruit is like loading yourself with thirty grams of sugar. For citrus fruit juice (discouraged in diabetes), four ounces, or half a cup, should come out to approximately fifteen grams.

Vegetables as Essentials in the Diet

Vegetables are vital to a healthy diet. Half of your dinner plate should be filled with vegetables. By so doing, you will know that your diet is providing the essential nutrients and fiber and keeping your weight within good range. Since vegetable food items are nutrient dense, the healthy elements will be high compared to the calorie content. Vegetables are usually easy to prepare, are readily available from any grocery store, and can be either cooked or eaten raw. Can it get any easier?

In the past, patients did not have to consider nonstarch vegetables when calculating grams of carbohydrates. Today, however, it has almost become a way of life. We have to keep an eye on the carbohydrates we eat because carbohydrates are the same thing as sugar. Diabetes, after all, involves harmful amounts of sugar in the circulatory system. Try eating three cups of nonstarch raw vegetables (the equivalent of fifteen grams of carbohydrates) or one and a half cups of cooked vegetables.

Diabetes and Dairy Products

Dairy products often have carbohydrates, protein, and fat. They also contain calcium, vitamin D, and other important vitamins and minerals. Low-fat dairy products help to cut the intake of saturated fats and cholesterol. When you buy these products in the grocery store, read the label to find the number of grams of carbohydrates in each serving. Eight ounces of milk has about twelve to fifteen grams of carbohydrates in it. Skim milk products like buttermilk may have much less. Hot cocoa and drink powders with artificial sweeteners or an eight-ounce container of yogurt can also be considered. In fact, all of the above dairy products can be included in the diabetic's diet.

A Glance at Simple Sugars

Simple sugars, another form of carbohydrates, can cause a quick spike in blood sugar. Taking fifteen grams of simple carbohydrates is recommended for low blood sugar. Fifteen grams of sugar is equivalent to two tablespoons of table sugar, one tablespoon of honey, four ounces of fruit juice, or eight ounces of nonfat milk. Nondiet sodas have a lot of simple sugar—around three tablespoons in a single twelve-ounce can. Corn syrups with high levels of fructose are also frequently being used in various food items and can cause a major increase in blood sugar levels after about five to ten minutes. Eating a lot of ketchup, which can be packed with sugar that often goes unnoticed by the consumer, can result in irregular amounts of blood glucose.

With all of these warnings, it is important that you stay mindful of everything you eat so you can determine what works for you. There may be hidden carbohydrate contents in some of the foods you eat, which can be dangerous if you don't pay attention to them.

Here is a good way to catch your carbs in the act: Just about any substance that ends in the suffix *-ose* is a sugar compound. As you may have noticed, sugar forms are labeled as *sucrose, dextrose, fructose, maltose,* and *lactose.* Carbohydrates are like thieves who can run but cannot hide!

Record your food intake religiously, including the estimated carbohydrate content, as well as the doses of insulin you take every day. This is how you can develop a sense of what you are taking in and form habits that are good for your health.

The Truth about Alcohol

Alcohol does not raise blood sugar levels all by itself. In fact, pure alcohol reduces the amount of sugar the liver produces, thereby reducing blood sugar levels. It is recommended that diabetics always eat something when drinking alcoholic beverages to prevent any possible reactions related to very low blood sugar. As well, sometimes alcohol is mixed with sweet mixers and juices for dilutive purposes, which is something you need to consider.

Below is a list of fruit drinks and their respective carbohydrate amounts:

- Strawberry daiquiri (twelve ounces)—thirty-six grams
- Margarita (twelve ounces)—forty-eight grams
- Piña colada (twelve ounces)—forty-eight grams
- Fuzzy navel (twelve ounces)—forty-two grams
- Vodka martini (four ounces)—forty grams

If you drink, understand that the above drinks have different effects depending on your blood glucose levels. For instance, beer has more carbohydrates than wine.

Drinking a tiny amount of alcohol is generally good for you. Avoid getting carried away, though, as brain and liver cells can die as a result. A glass of wine at dinner can aid in removing many causes of heart disease. If you are including alcohol as part of your diet, you should remember these simple benchmarks:

- One drink serving is equal to around twelve ounces of beer, four ounces of wine, or one and half ounces of distilled spirits.

- If you consume alcohol every day, the calories must be noted in the meal plan. If you are concerned about gaining weight, alcohol may be substituted for servings of fat. A serving of alcohol is equal to two servings of fat.
- Be mindful of the calories and carbohydrates contained in any mixers or juices being used.

THE STRENGTH OF PROTEINS

While there may be a formula for calculating the minimum amount of protein to include in a low-fat, high-carb diet, many physicians believe there really isn't a straightforward calculation that diabetics can use to measure protein. They simply suggest that diabetics eat reasonable amounts of high-protein foods they enjoy, such as fish, poultry, pork, beef, and eggs. It is also advisable that you eat until you are satisfied, not until you are stuffed.

The quality of the protein you eat is just as vital as its quantity. Let's take a look at the complete contents of protein, which include reasonable amounts of all nine essential amino acids. You can get all of these amino acids from poultry, meat, fish, eggs, dairy products, and other animal foods. However, grains and legumes do not contain sufficient amounts of protein.

Plant foods also have the complete set of amino acids required in the diet, but in most, at least one amino acid is present in less than the recommended quantity. Grains, which are low in lysine, and beans, which are low in sulfur amino acids like methionine and cysteine, have reduced amounts of proteins.

If a person fails to get enough amino acids from the plant sources they usually eat, or if they do not eat animal foods, they can still get the necessary amino acids from a combination of plant-derived foods like peanuts, seeds, legumes, and whole grains.

Eggs are often believed to be unhealthy because of their high cholesterol content, but you can include them in moderate amounts. This is because of their low GI ranking and their high content of vitamins D, B, and E, together with the minerals calcium, zinc, iron, potassium, and magnesium. Egg yolks get their yellow color from carotenoids called lutein and zeaxanthin. These molecules can protect the eyes from macular degeneration. Macular degeneration is a disease in which the retina of the eye begins to degenerate, leading to an age-related loss of vision.

When you consume adequate amounts of protein, your sugar levels can also be kept right. As a diabetic you can always get the right amount of proteins and other nutrients if you pay attention to what's in your food.

You can get vitamin D from eggs, butter, cheese, and fish. It is suggested that you consume vitamin D in moderate amounts, supplemented with calcium and phosphorus. Remember the protein-packed soy foods, which are rich in Vitamin D, and include them in your meals at least twice a week. Stick to organic meats and eggs for the long term if you really think protein shortage is a major problem with your diet.

As a diabetic, avoiding unhealthy foods is a significant step toward dealing with the symptoms of the disease. Approaching your diabetes from a dietary standpoint usually depends on how fervent and dedicated you really are as a patient. Finally, always make modifications to your diet based on recommendations from a health professional.

· 10 ·

Pain Management for the Diabetic

$\mathscr{P}$ain is an unfortunate and unavoidable consequence of diabetes. Insulin shots, injections, blood sugar testing—all of these modes of treatment, combined with the complications of diabetes itself, can cause pain for the diabetic. This is why routine pain therapy and management is such an important part of the diabetic's life.

WHAT TO DO ABOUT PAIN

When you are ready to fight pain effectively, two things must be understood: how you define your own pain, and how you plan to deal with it. Perhaps you already have an idea about what pain is and what the common remedies are, but first you have to recognize the causes of painful experiences as they relate to the mind and body. If this isn't done, you may be missing, or misunderstanding, the roots of your diabetic problem.

Only in recent years has modern medicine begun to unlock the mysteries of pain. The many mechanisms involved must be understood in order for us to get a handle on diabetes holistically.

Try to imagine pain. Anyone can. Pain, especially acute pain, is an inevitable and universal part of being human. In the words of Marcel Proust, "Pain is a tyrant whose commands everyone is impelled to obey." Even though pain is often associated with the negative aspects of life, it can also protect your health. Pain is the human body's alarm system. Evolution has given us this mechanism to warn us against suffering and injury. When the injury is internal, pain can be a detriment to vital functions, such as eating and sleeping.

161

GETTING RID OF PAIN: IT'S EITHER NOW OR NEVER

A red light goes on in your body when you have acute pain, which is a warning sign of a minor or major injury. This convinces the diabetic to seek treatment.

Pain serves as a daily reminder that the human body has purposes, among which is to save itself from harm. As a whole, the human body is remarkably resilient considering what it is made of. Our first line of defense is our skin, a miraculous organ with about twenty square feet of surface area. Comprised of layer after layer of microscopic cells, it shields the body's inner workings from destructive microorganisms and other contaminants. It also contains a meshwork of millions of sensory nerves, which give us a sense of touch and allow us to avoid things that could cause serious harm.

Without a sense of pain, our ability to pinpoint when and where damage has occurred would be virtually nonexistent. An illness that lacks painful symptoms can be especially insidious.

Pain is exceptionally subjective; a doctor cannot diagnose what kind of pain you are feeling any more than he or she can read your mind. Only the sufferer can describe the type or degree of his or her pain experience. As a result, definitions and descriptions of pain differ among individuals. Chronic pain is long-term pain; a sufferer of chronic pain can expect a lifetime of unpleasant experiences.

As pain is an intriguing subject, doctors have challenged themselves to try and understand it better. It is not a disease in and of itself, but rather a symptom that you could never see under a microscope or find evidence of in a blood test. It isn't just an event like a heart attack, which concentrates on a single organ or system. Neither is it wholly a psychological phenomenon like a mental illness. Pain can be all of these things and more, owing to its subjective nature. It is universal but paradoxically inconsistent from person to person; feeling another's pain is a *physio*logical and *psycho*logical impossibility. A level of pain that one person can simply shrug off may leave another crying like an infant.

"Pain is what the patient says it is." This is one of the definitions many health care professionals use to explain what pain really is. Various feelings are involved in the entire pain experience. Just like emotions, pain is a mixture of various aspects that differ depending on person and magnitude. This is why diabetic pain should be approached holistically at all times.

PATHWAYS OF PAIN

The Enlightenment philosopher René Descartes, the man who coined the famous phrase, "I think, therefore I am," also said that pain is like a pathway.

It is a unique sensation, apart from the common senses like sight, smell, and touch. It is in a league of its own. Descartes' view is that several threads or fibers form the nerves that run through the skin and the relevant parts of the brain. A metaphor has been conceived to portray Descartes' thoughts: a rope and a bell.

This perception seems accurate at first glance, as pain apparently begins traveling from a narrow origin and accumulates in another location of the body. However, pain does not travel along a single path but along two main routes: the central nervous system, which includes the brain and spinal cord, and the peripheral nervous system, which encompasses all the other nerves. These main routes branch off into many other pathways, intersections, detours, and loops. Pain is a complicated area of medical research that carries many secrets that have yet to be uncovered.

Pain is not static but rather a complicated process. It can move from point to point through various paths, manifesting in different ways at different intersections. Recently, scientists have shed some light on how neuronal organization is altered by pain. Since diabetic patients tend to suffer from unexpected bouts of pain, knowing how pain works can help gain the edge against diabetes.

THE INTENSIVE THEORY

Long before Descartes, the philosopher Aristotle had his own theories on pain. He described pain as a magnified sensation of any sort; that is, pain is an excessive sensitivity, largely pertaining to touch and temperature. In the nineteenth century, scientists expanded this theory to include all the senses.

Aristotle's theory that pain is like a magnifying glass is also consistent with the subjective nature of pain. A magnifying glass not only magnifies but also distorts, making objects in the center appear larger and objects at the edges appear smaller. So everyone's internal magnifying glass focuses in a different location. An unbearable sensation for one may be easily tolerable to another, and vice versa.

If you suffer from foot ulcers, you might tolerate the experience without any pain medications, while another diabetic must constantly take medications to simply function normally. This may even change as time goes on. At one moment, an individual may feel as if he or she could withstand a particular pain experience forever, but at the next moment, the same sensation may bring the patient to his or her knees.

This emphasizes the fact that the mind has the final say over how pain is experienced: diabetics can subjectively experience the same physical experience in holistically different ways. With the mind and body connection firmly established, we now have a new theory in hand suggesting that it may be possible to fool the mind into ignoring pain altogether.

The fact that your emotional state determines the impact that pain has on you corroborates this theory. When we say that someone is in a good mood, we imply that he or she is feeling no pain and that such a happy person would not be bothered by pain nearly as much. On the other hand, feelings of anxiety in response to pain can alter a person's psychology to such an extent that what would normally be considered minor discomfort may be almost unbearable. These two opposing scenarios suggest that pain can be managed and controlled with the right psychological approach.

These are not the only theories that shed light on the phenomenon of pain, but for now, we will stick to these two. In the next section, we will discuss the relationship between pain and diabetes.

THE CONNECTION BETWEEN PAIN AND DIABETES

Juvenile and adult-onset diabetes are the most common types of the illness, with around 800,000 new cases every year. These forms of diabetes can damage organs like the kidneys, heart, and bowels. Digestion is impeded, leading to heart disease and the slow destruction of the nervous system. This accumulated damage to the body's systems is the culprit behind the most common pain symptom of diabetes: diabetic neuropathy.

Diabetic neuropathy typically leaves the sufferer unable to walk without excruciating pain. Some diabetics suffering from neuropathy have described it as feeling like their feet are on fire. Their feet become so incredibly sensitive to pain that even socks can cause intense discomfort. The only way to avoid the pain is to avoid walking altogether. The psychological consequences of this can be devastating. Crippling pain, combined with a sense of helplessness, can leave a diabetic completely lost and unable to cope.

This makes us ponder even deeper the subjective nature of pain and its relation to the sufferer's mood: does having a smile on your face and having a positive outlook relieve pain?

For many years, researchers have been trying to devise just the right scale for measuring pain. The Bennett model is one such attempt, devised by Dr. Gary Bennett of Allegheny University's Department of Neurology. His model of neuropathic pain is intended to help shed light on painful disorders like diabetic neuropathy and aid in the development of treatments.

Developing such a model initially involved finding and applying objective means of measuring pain responses. For instance, the sciatic nerve can be tied with a suture to produce a measurable form of neuropathic pain. The von Frey hair is a tool dating back to the late nineteenth century and is still in common use. It consists of a nylon strand of a specific thickness that is pressed against the skin until the strand bends. This simple tool measures a direct correlation between pain and the application of force. Thermal sensory testing is another method which involves the use of heat and cold to measure pain. Applying a metal disk such as a Peltier thermode to the finger and then heating it to a precise temperature allows the researcher to find the exact point at which a subject's pain response causes them to withdraw their hand.

As neuropathic pain can result from injury anywhere in the nervous system, physicians need various methods to detect and measure it. The autonomic nervous system (ANS) regulates blood pressure and heart rate. It changes skin temperature by contracting the small blood vessels. Applying this knowledge brings us to the use of a Doppler scanner, which measures skin temperature as an indicator of blood flow. It can scan the extremities and display blood flow in the form of a color-coded chart, ranging from red (flow increase) to blue (flow decrease). The Doppler scanner reveals how blood flow is affected by reactions to environmental changes. For example, being startled by a loud noise or holding your breath means the ANS is hard at work.

In the past, doctors typically thought of pain as a universal symptom and were blind to its subjective nature. In modern times, it is properly recognized not as a single symptom but as a category of various symptoms. There are many different and distinct kinds of pain, and understanding this is of high importance for both diagnosis and holistic treatment of diabetes.

THE ROAD TO TREATING NEUROPATHY

The interesting studies discussed so far only describe neuropathy in terms of symptoms from a layperson's viewpoint. Neuropathy manifests itself as an altered sensitivity in the nerves at the fringes of the peripheral nervous system, particularly those found in the hands and feet. Diabetes starves these nerves, compromising our ability to sense what genuinely constitutes pain. Skin contact in the nerve damage site can exaggerate your physical perception of pain. This could scare you enough to cause an overreaction to your symptoms, since it makes you feel better to be safe than sorry.

With the root cause of neuropathic pain firmly established, it is plain as day that the key to treating this crippling condition is to target the nerves themselves, not merely the afflicted areas. This is typically accomplished by testing the sufferer's reaction to an anesthetic like lidocaine. If lidocaine successfully alleviates your chronic pain, then you can be prescribed similar medications in the long term.

One type of drug that may be administered is an oral version of an antiarrhythmia medication, which soothes the nerves, prevents their irregular activity, and functions as an analgesic. Should this be insufficient in alleviating symptoms, an anticonvulsant may be administered to prevent the erratic nerve signals. Commonly used anticonvulsants include the following:

- Carbamazepine (Tegretol)
- Gabapentin (Neurontin)
- Clonazepan (Klonopin)
- Phenytoin (Dilantin)
- Valproic acid (Depakote)

Calcium channel blockers have also been shown to be a potential means for combating the symptoms of neuropathy. These medications include verapamil, diltiazem, nifedipine, nicardipine, and nimodipine. By changing the flow of calcium to and from cell membranes, and thus the flow of electrical signals, researchers believe that these drugs may be able to relieve pain.

N-methyl d-aspartate (NMDA) inhibitors are another subject that researchers study like a hawk. It is believed that NMDA receptors play a role in the malfunctioning of the nervous system that leads to neuropathy. The ability to block these receptors may be the secret to preventing acute pain from becoming chronic pain. NMDA inhibitors have been available for years, but drugs in this category powerful enough to have a positive effect on pain typically have a number of negative side effects. Pain relief centers still use a mild NMDA inhibitor known as dextromethorphan, an ingredient commonly found in Robitussin cough syrup. NMDA is also useful in the field of addiction rehabilitation as a means of ending a patient's reliance on narcotics. While the effects of NMDA and drugs intended to block such receptors are still under study, it is possible that this category of drug will have a promising future in pain relief.

DEPRESSION AND PAIN

Neuropathic pain can also lead to depression, yet there is very little overlap between drugs for pain relief and drugs for depression. Dr. Scott Fishman has therefore advocated a divide-and-conquer strategy to deal with the two issues as separate and independent conditions.

Some antidepressants have been shown to combat nerve pain, including the tricyclic drugs amitriptyline (Elavil), nortriptyline (Pamelor), desipramine

(Norpramin), and imipramine (Tofranil). The Prozac-like selective serotonin reuptake inhibitors (SSRI) do not appear to moonlight as painkillers. This may be because these particular drugs don't inhibit seizures. Depression itself can trigger pain, and Prozac and similar drugs tend to have fewer side effects than the tricyclic antidepressants, so SSRI drugs may be the best option for someone who suffers from both depression and neuropathic pain.

Diverse remedies for managing pain are in common use today. Since ancient times, people have been discovering and developing various means for reducing or eliminating pain. From this point on, we will discuss the different regimens you can turn to besides the typical pain medications.

PAIN IN THE MUSCLES AND JOINTS

Diabetics may experience sensations that make them feel unpleasant, such as tightness in the muscles or pain and swelling in the joints. It may be wise not to regard these feelings as simple, curable pain, but rather as expressions of other conditions related to diabetes that can be reversed.

If your body weight is far outside the ideal BMI range, losing weight can help alleviate pain symptoms. High levels of insulin can cause joint inflammation and lead to wear and tear. Switching to a vegetarian diet can help solve this issue.

The most common form of degenerative joint disease is osteoarthritis, in which the protective cartilage that cushions the force of bone against bone is degraded. Cartilage also allows for stability and flexibility, working with the ligaments and tendons that connect joint structures. If untreated, this condition can leave you crippled. Bear in mind that as the years go by, the finger joints age and tend to swell and stiffen, especially in the morning.

Activity patterns and accompanying pain experiences should be noted and correlated. This way, pain-producing behaviors can be recognized and avoided. There is an old joke where a man tells his doctor, "It hurts when I do this." The doctor replies, "Then stop doing that!" This might get laughs, but it is valid advice in these circumstances. Diabetics with osteoarthritis can benefit from exercise, but again, repetitive strain on joints prone to osteoarthritis should be avoided if possible.

There may also be the presence of red and swollen joints, especially if the condition is persistent and symmetrical. Specifically, the same joints on both sides of the body are affected, indicating either rheumatoid or septic (infectious) arthritis. Depending on location and exposure, these symptoms may also be the result of Lyme disease, an illness transmitted by tick bites.

Whatever the case, an actual diagnosis should remain the duty of a doctor, not yours.

Non-weight-bearing joints, such as the elbows and shoulders, can be checked for their range of motion and assessed for any restriction in movement or movement-associated pain. The surrounding tissue and shape of the joint itself should also be checked out for any irregularities. A change in condition should be treated with special care, and massages and exercise may also be beneficial. You should, however, consult a physician to ensure that any measures you take will not exacerbate the problem.

GOOD PAIN, BAD PAIN, AND EXERCISE

When you begin an exercise routine, a trivial amount of stiffness and soreness is perfectly normal. These occur because unused muscles and joints are seeing action for the first time in a long while. We have already come to the conclusion that pain is the body's way of warning itself about injury, but it can also be a benign side effect of strenuous activity.

Question: how can you tell the difference between "bad" pain and "good" pain?

Good pain is a slight dull ache or soreness in a muscle, or perhaps a minor stiffness surrounding a joint that goes away after a few days. It can also disappear following a good long soak in a warm bath. As you get more accustomed to the activity, the pain will diminish.

Bad pain is sharp or sudden and continues after halting the activity. This can indicate either a problem with the joint involved or an injury. If the pain is severe or persistent, or the joint is red and swollen, you should see a doctor immediately.

MANAGEMENT OF DIABETIC NERVE PAIN

Diabetic nerve pain at times tends to make a sore life for almost all diabetics, and researchers around the globe are currently working on this issue. Diabetes associated with nerve pain can truly take a toll on the circulatory capabilities of the body. You shouldn't be negligent about this pain, but take steps at the first opportunity.

It is essential to learn the secrets of how to take charge of the tyranny of diabetic nerve pain. Here is an easy-to-follow pathway that can keep diabetic nerve pain at bay:

- To alleviate the level of diabetic nerve pain experienced by a patient, some sort of physical activity is helpful but shouldn't be too exhausting. Regular walking is a good idea to keep your mind away from the pain. It also leads to proper circulation in the body.
- Drinking lots of water can boost your resistance to pain. Without water flowing through your digestive and circulatory system, toxins hang around and cause harm.
- Glucose levels should be checked regularly. If your diabetes is controllable, then checking your sugars is the best way to avoid diabetic nerve pain.
- Application of diabetic creams can give the diabetic patient a respite from the painful effects of diabetes.
- Foods rich with the omega-3 fatty acids are highly effective in controlling diabetic nerve pain.
- Vitamin D products like milk can help a lot to curb the levels of diabetic nerve pain.
- Soda, carbonated drinks, and caffeine drinks should be removed from the diabetic's menu. These foods are not all that nutritious, but they can make pain worse. Hence they are better avoided altogether.
- Eating cold-water fish regularly is a good way of controlling diabetic nerve pain, as these fish are rich in omega-3 fatty acids.

ALTERNATIVE METHODS

While the following methods may not cure diabetes, they can come in handy when targeting pain and stress caused by metabolic functions (such as oxidation) or hormones that have the opposite effects of the action of insulin in the body. Reducing these stresses can have a good result on glucose levels and can also aid in treating the neuropathic pain caused by diabetes.

Acupuncture

Hailing from China, this ancient practice is based on the principle that good health and well-being require a free flow of energy (qi) throughout one's body and between one's organs. Qi flows through a network of energy channels, or "meridians," in the body. An acupuncturist inserts a very slender sterilized needle into key points to stimulate these meridians and balance the flow of qi. This relieves pain and promotes healing in the process. If the concept of needle pricking shocks you, reap the benefits of acupuncture via other methods: heat and cold application, pressure, small gold or silver pellets, electrical stimulation, and modern-day low-intensity lasers.

It is certainly tempting to look into some acupuncture treatment procedures that work miracles, but it also essential to have a complete grasp on the subject before we actually take a tour of acupuncture as a treatment for diabetes. Acupuncture is accredited globally as an effective procedure that establishes a perfect sense of balance between bodily functions. As a matter of fact, there may be a number of causes responsible for a severe or imbalance in the body. Genetic disorders are consistent with this theory, since they can cause severe stress or unwanted anxiety levels. Acupuncture therapies are carried out in an attempt to synchronize all the body systems.

Treatment Procedures of Acupuncture Pertaining to Diabetes

If you really need acupuncture therapy, you would be introduced to the procedure based on the five-element theory. Five-element acupuncture is an accredited procedure for diabetes and is known to provide positive results in any kind of disease. The five elements of acupuncture are fire, earth, metal, wood, and water. This is the ancient, down-to-earth form of acupuncture. It is believed that these five elements are empowered to establish a new wave of energy in the human body, which will help to create a never-ending harmony in a person. With this five-element acupuncture procedure, cholesterol and triglyceride levels can be kept in check. Ultimately, you get much better control of glucose. That's the reason why most doctors in the world refer patients for acupuncture at some point in their career.

Pulse Diagnosis Treatment

Pulse diagnosis treatment is a reputable treatment in the field of acupuncture. It is a very comprehensive technique. When it comes to effectiveness, this special technique is really amazing, and it is generally practiced in sessions with an acupuncture veteran. The power of pulse diagnosis is fascinating, at least in terms of strengthening the energy level of a diabetic patient. That is why pulse diagnosis patients hardly ever revert to traditional medical treatments. This is an ancient form of treatment that is highly useful. It is also an established practice in ayurvedic medicine.

To begin with, pulse diagnosis investigates your health by reading your pulse. Then the practitioner comes up with a list of options for you. Pulse diagnosis procedures for diabetes not only consider your pulse but also your current body temperature, moisture, swelling, and any existing chronic disease besides diabetes. Genuine pulse diagnosis treatments should focus on the traditional "twelve points" of the human body. Stress management techniques to control the nervous system and appease nerve pain can also be applied. Soothing background music creates an ideal therapeutic atmosphere for the diabetic patient getting acupuncture treatment.

Low glycemic foods and a low-fat diet are advised. As a matter of fact, consumption of food has a lot to do with controlling the capacity of a diabetes patient. Even after complete acupuncture therapy, the entire procedure can go awry if you don't maintain a good amount of control over your diet. The treatment must be a good and healthy combination of acupuncture visits and disciplined lifestyle.

Smoking and alcohol consumption should be strictly avoided because they are detrimental to the diabetic patient. The entire treatment and the efforts of the patient would go to waste in the absence of restraints on smoking and drinking. In order to obtain the best results, one should cease these two addictions for good.

Experts believe that meditation and prayer are important aspects of the acupuncture process. These two rituals are more than enough to establish an atmosphere of calmness and poise in the mind of the diabetic patient. They create an attitude in the mind of the diabetic patient that convinces him or her to fight back. They give a diabetic patient the power to win against diabetes and live a regular, happy life.

Biofeedback

This simple technique focuses on stress management through relaxation and instructions for how diabetic patients can respond better to neuropathic pain. Biofeedback trains the subject to control the flow of blood to one hand, the tension in muscles throughout the body, or even heart rate in order to reach a state of deep relaxation. This reduces stress hormone levels, blood pressure, and pain, and can even diminish the effects of certain heart and lung diseases.

Guided Imagery

Guided imagery is another helpful relaxation technique in which the subject centers his or her mind on positive healing images. The imagery is designed to produce a relaxation response and a targeted immune reaction. For example, guided imagery may be used to help strengthen the immune system against cancerous cells. Through the work of pioneers like Dr. Bernie Seigel and Dr. Carl Simonton, this technique has been used along with other methods of treatment to preserve the right metabolism levels, to prevent the enlargement of tumors, and to attain a better sense of well-being and quality of life.

Despite having been in use for decades, scientific backing for the effectiveness of guided imagery remains a challenge.

Hypnosis

Once merely a part of magic shows and other entertainment, today hypnotism serves the field of medicine as much as it serves to delight and amaze audiences. Its means of operation are not fully understood, but it is very powerful against postoperative discomfort and as a form of anesthesia for a whole host of surgeries: brain surgery, tooth extractions, thyroidectomies, appendectomies, heart surgery, caesarean sections, and the list goes on. Clinics use it to care for burn patients while their dressings are changed.

Hypnosis has also been applied with success to other illnesses, as reported in several cases of severe depression and anxiety, as well as for diabetic neuropathic pain and diabetic blindness. One such patient was also suffering from diabetic gastroparesis, a slowed digestive response caused by nerve injury. This condition, previously managed by narcotic pain drugs, is associated with distended bowels resulting from severe constipation.

The patient receiving hypnosis therapy is asked to close his or her eyes to mentally visualize a house or some other appeasing place. Vivid imagery supplied by the imagination aids the process. If done with care and expertise, the patient soon falls into a deep sleep or trance. This causes a positive response that can help alleviate pain.

Studies on the means by which hypnosis produces these results suggest that the subject's brain waves are altered during hypnotic episodes. One theory holds that the trance initiated by hypnosis activates pain-killing parts of the brain. Another theory says hypnosis disconnects pain sensations from the mind's "receiving antennae."

Though cases in which hypnosis has proved effective in pain therapy are well documented, the fact remains that not everyone can be successfully hypnotized. According to Dr. Maxwell Shapiro, a well-known psychologist and hypnotherapist at the Massachusetts General Hospital, people with active imaginations, the kind that can become absorbed in a movie, book, television program, or other activity, are highly receptive to hypnotic procedures.

The success of hypnosis therapy on diabetics also hinges on three further factors. First is the patient's motivation and ability to establish rapport with the doctor. Second, patients have to trust the physician's skill and ability to hypnotize them. Third, the patient must understand that hypnosis will lead to a positive change. An expert hypnotherapist has no need for complex equipment; even the traditional swinging pendulum is not a requirement. A skilled hypnotist can hypnotize a patient using his or her voice alone. Incredible!

MORE BEHAVIORAL TREATMENTS

Behavioral medicine assesses the mental impact of pain on your life. Using this information, solutions for restoring lost functionality can be implemented along with support healing. Since chronic pain may last a lifetime, behavioral specialists help by enabling you to cope and separate the painful experiences from your life.

Behavioral therapists do not accept that the mind and body are wholly separate in function, playing it safe not to lead the diabetic into thinking the pain is imaginary and is therefore purely psychological. However, pain can have psychological roots, particularly stress and tension. These conditions fuel the fire for pain and may also trigger new pains. The most effective means for combating these bouts of pain is through relaxation techniques.

Pain and relaxation are like two opposing forces. They coexist but constantly oppose one another, almost the same way oil and water do. You must develop good balancing strategies to shatter the tension caused by everyday issues. Relaxation is one such mechanism. Apart from the methods we have discussed before, breathing exercises are a simple relaxation technique that can be carried out without extra help.

The effectiveness of simple breathing exercises against stress and pain has been a hot research topic for years. Breathing has a direct link to the body's alarm systems. Think about the horror we feel at the slightest hint of suffocation, when we are reminded of our own breathing. Hold your breath for about twenty seconds and note the feeling. This same mechanism triggers anxiety, agitation, high blood pressure, and rapid heart rate in response to fear, triggering panic attacks. Improper breathing can have any number of negative effects on your life. Regulating the way you breathe can reverse these effects and even set a positive change in motion.

Take an extremely deep breath in and out, slowly and easily. Like all other basic human functions, deep relaxed breathing is a collaboration of mind and body that wakes up the autonomic nervous system and allows us to feel calm.

Air is generally drawn into two areas of the lungs, but when we are stressed or anxious, there is a tendency to breathe in short gulps, pulling air into the relatively shallow chest or thoracic region. These quick gulps of air stimulate parts of the autonomic nervous system, preparing the body's "fight or flight" response. The nervous system then demands the production of adrenaline, which speeds up both heart rate and breathing rate, increases blood pressure, and shifts the flow of blood from the organs to the muscles.

The antidote for stress and mental tension is deeper and slower breathing, also known as abdominal breathing. It draws with force from deep within the diaphragm, preventing the fight-or-flight response and supporting the alternate response called "feed or breed." Through this, anxiety and stress are counterbalanced as your heart rate slows and blood pressure goes down. One way to practice deep breathing is by lying on your back and placing your hands over your chest and abdomen as you breathe. During this time, you should be able to take in more air and subsequently relax both mind and muscle.

Deep breathing is not the only relaxation method at your disposal. Visualization and introspection can also improve physical awareness and replace pain sensations with a warm, relaxed feeling.

Additionally, there is the technique known as autogenic relaxation. The patient is asked to close his or her eyes while focusing on a part of the body—the arms, for instance—and to explain how it feels in terms of weight, temperature, and so forth. As the patient explores these feelings, the physician will offer a relaxing phrase for them to repeat, such as "I feel really quiet." During this process, the doctor may also monitor and record the patient's temperature and ask what images he or she sees mentally. Enhancing physical awareness and generating warmth in the targeted area in this fashion allows a diabetic to relax and relieve pain anytime, anywhere. Amazing, isn't it?

Relaxation training is a vital aspect of the treatments offered by various clinics and institutions. Specialists teach their patients about relaxing during a busy day using the "quieting response." This therapeutic procedure trains you to relax at all times, even if you are unable to do deep breathing or autogenic exercises during work. Writing therapy, biofeedback, cognitive psychotherapy in minor doses, and possibly hypnosis may be used.

A diabetic's personal recognition and conducive attitude toward pain and how it meshes or clashes with their life is vital to successful behavioral therapy. This is essential to any treatment, and a positive attitude toward a solution can provide benefits regardless of whether there is an intrinsic power to heal. A negative outlook toward a treatment can put the kibosh on its potential benefits or even cause harm.

PUTTING A KNIFE TO IT: SURGICAL OPTIONS

Somewhere along the way, back pain may add itself to the list of symptoms a diabetic endures. Physicians may recommend surgical treatment rather than medication and relaxation techniques. Is such a drastic step necessary, or even beneficial?

Whether just a symptom of another ailment or a condition on its own, lower back pain has been documented throughout history and still leaves us with many mysteries. In the nineteenth century, lower back pain was taken as a disease caused by an "irritated spine" or trauma. When the Social Security system was first introduced, lower back pain became known as a symptom of poor work conditions and thus a reason for workers' compensation. From that point onward, the focus shifted from remedies to the elimination of the "disease." In 1934, herniation of the spinal discs was discovered as one cause of lower back pain, giving rise to the possibility of surgical treatment.

If as a diabetic you suffer from chronic back pain, you may have already considered the idea of a surgical fix, especially if your X-ray or MRI (magnetic resonance imaging) results show worn or otherwise abnormal discs and joints. This physical aspect of back pain means that surgery can be carried out to prevent damage to the discs or spinal cord. It also serves as an option for pain relief when you are at the end of your rope.

Typical forms of surgery for back pain include laminectomy, discectomy, and spinal fusion, focusing on structural repairs to discs or vertebrae. Depending on the patient, these surgeries may be done as separate operations or in combination.

A laminectomy removes the lamina, a part of the vertebra, to relieve pressure on the spinal cord. Only one lamina is usually taken out, but if multiple laminae need to be removed, the procedure will involve a spinal fusion. The sole purpose of spinal fusion is to prevent abnormal movement of the spine by binding two vertebrae together, usually using a bone graft taken from another part of the body. On its own, a spinal fusion may be performed to correct instability in the spine, typically caused by injury or disease.

A discectomy is performed to remove a herniated or ruptured disc. Herniation means that the disc's "jelly" interior has been squeezed out through the harder outer layer. This material is typically kept away from other tissues by the disc's outer layer, and it inflames the bones and nerves when it comes in contact with them. Surgery can clear out this leakage. However, disc herniation often dissipates of its own accord, making it possible to recover even without surgery or direct intervention. The same can be said about lower back pain, which despite the prevalence of surgical options, may subside via common pain relief methods.

The problem here is that surgical operations for the diabetic don't offer a pain relief guarantee. In fact, invasive surgery can lead to further trauma, potentially adding new chronic pain symptoms or making existing ones worse.

HEADACHES AND SO MUCH MORE

Headaches in all their different guises have long been recognized as symptomatic of underlying conditions. Tension headaches, migraines, sinus headaches, hangover headaches, eyestrain headaches, caffeine withdrawal headaches—one could go on.

Unsurprisingly, headaches are a recurring issue in diabetes. With all we have discussed so far, what can you do to hold back the pain or remove the headache altogether?

On the medication front is a class of drugs called triptans. Second-generation triptans have been recently discovered to be helpful against headaches, and unlike most migraine drugs, they can make the headache disappear entirely. The new generation of triptans tones down related symptoms, such as nausea and sensitivity to light and sound, all without sedative side effects.

Natural herbs like feverfew are believed to help alleviate chronic pain. However, physicians don't usually recommend feverfew because it is not yet fully understood. The plant's holistic effectiveness and side effects also remain as one of the most profound medical mysteries.

ANOTHER OPTION: PHYSICAL THERAPY

The time may come when a patient suffering from chronic pain loses hope and stops going to their physician for treatment. In the long run, these diabetics tend to feel that no treatment can help their pain experience. "So, why bother trying?" they ask.

What they don't understand is that there is still one more option: physical therapy.

Physical therapy (PT) is all about increasing your functioning and improving the quality of your life through movement. Growing public acceptance of physical therapy has made it a state-of-the-art option for pain treatment.

Physical therapists teach their patients how to manage pain rather than prescribing treatments that will sooner or later fail. You may be told on your first visit that PT does not work for every individual, but a positive viewpoint is vital to its success. Diabetics also have to accept that the responsibility of managing their pain falls on them, not on some hypothetical miracle cure.

Preliminary visits will include physical assessments to analyze the patient's condition. Gait, posture, sitting tolerance, flexibility, and muscle strength are all studied, and the level of pain is measured accordingly. The results of these tests determine what the prescribed systematic plan will be for the future.

If you are a physical therapy patient, you may be prescribed a regimen including the following:

- Sitting for about fifteen minutes a day, with one minute added for each day that passes

- Icing the back four times a day for a minimum of twenty minutes total
- Walking ten minutes twice a day, with one minute added for each day that passes
- Pelvic tilting or bending three times a day

Traction is an alternative method that blocks generalized back discomfort, especially when there are signs of disc degeneration. A traction device tugs on the lower back, gently pulling the vertebrae apart and relieving pressure on the nerve roots responsible for the pain. Lumbar traction may lead to relaxed muscles surrounding the spine and an opening of the space between vertebral joints. There is evidence that reducing the electrical activity of pain nerves in the lumbar region in this way can reduce pain to a certain extent. Traction alone cannot cure diabetic pain, but it can take away the stress on your back very efficiently. This is a long-lasting pain relief option, among many others, that you might want to consider as a diabetic.

· 11 ·

Staying Motivated

*W*hen faced with diabetes—yours or a loved one's—you must stay motivated at all times. You may need to develop methods for coping even when your situation seems desperate. Understand, this disease *can* be licked through motivation and hard work.

We have already talked about diet, emotions, weight, medications, and other kinds of treatment regimens, but the success of any plan depends on one person: you. In a sense, you are the creative director of your own lifestyle and any changes you make. You are the one who must reflect on what works and what doesn't work in your treatment. You set your short- and long-term goals, and you are the one who will see the treatment through to the end.

The important thing to remember as you struggle through the trials and tribulations of your disease is that you are not helpless, and never will be, against diabetes. With the lessons you have learned already and those yet to come, you can win the fight against diabetes and its complications. So, let's continue with a few strategies to support you in living a healthier life as a diabetic.

HEALTH CARE PROFESSIONALS ARE THERE TO HELP YOU

One important step on this journey is establishing a close connection with your expert team composed of your primary physician, endocrinologist, nurse, educator, nutritionist, physical therapist, and so forth. Depending on the specifics of your condition, you may need to coordinate with other people you may not know but who are really there to help you. Build a good relationship with your health care professionals so that they can help you understand your disease and guide you as a patient. Once you have identified and established rapport with your health care experts, you need to stay focused on the goals you set together. Diabetes is a challenge, and one you may not succeed in unless you continue a healthy lifestyle and stay motivated.

We will be dealing with healthy diets and exercise in this chapter, along with behavioral factors and ways to make your experience as a diabetic more worthwhile.

MOTIVATION FOR EXERCISE AND WEIGHT LOSS

Losing weight and living free from diabetes is a struggle, even when armed with expert knowledge. Temptation is everywhere: on television, in public, and inside your refrigerator. If you spent your entire life prior to diabetes eating whatever you wanted, it may take time and practice to get used to the idea of a specialized diet, not to mention a great deal of self-control. View your diet as your best friend, not your enemy. This will be a strong step toward managing all the obstacles diabetes throws in your path.

Imagine yourself struggling to put on a pair of jeans this afternoon. Rewind to the year before, when you were struggling just to get off the couch because you spent hours in front of the TV and kept telling yourself you would get around to exercising later.

Picture yourself wearing a much smaller pair of jeans a year from today. Now imagine feeling a sense of well-being and increased energy because of it. Imagine yourself standing up from that couch and taking a walk. That possibility can turn into reality right now if you want it to. It might last only fifteen minutes the first day, but it is still a step toward good health. Exercise is not a "later" thing. It is very much a "now" thing. Every little bit helps: stretching, walking, anything that keeps you in motion and off the couch. Find your perfect exercise spot, somewhere you can work out without interruption. Above all, stay focused—the most important thing you need to work on is yourself!

Learning that you have diabetes is a life-altering experience. Diets, professional activities, and medications all appear to be intruders on what you previously considered "normal." It can seem like there is nothing you can do to improve things and that it is simply better to jump back on that couch and dive back into self-indulgence.

Where are you now as a diabetic? Where do you stand against your disease? You feel like there is something missing in your life, something that could be better, but what can you do?

As long as you can look at your life objectively and understand that you have room for improvements and opportunities, you have hope. With some dedication on your part, you can face this challenge and break through it.

Negativity is your foe. It makes you think you are truly helpless, that there is no hope in your future, that the road to happiness and the road to self-destruction are one and the same. Sift out these ideas from your mind and adopt a can-do mind-set. As long as you believe things can get better, it is very likely that they will.

A change has to come from both within and without. You can only change your health for the better if you change your overall outlook for the better. Do not be disheartened by stories of people who followed some miracle diet and ended up with a perfect physique. You are your own person, and your journey toward losing weight and improving your health will no doubt be just as unique as you are.

Do the research, read books about weight loss, and occasionally watch health shows on TV that have diabetes experts as guests. Get the fight against this disease started as soon as possible. Books and articles on dieting can provide valuable insight toward developing your own perfect strategy to achieve wellness, though you should always take the time and effort to verify your facts before you act on them. Consult with your nutritionist or physician. It seems like everyone these days has their own self-prescribed diet, so it is probably time you had one, too. Just walk into any bookstore and check out the wealth of diet-related material to get you started.

There's no time like the present—right here, right now—to commit to a healthier lifestyle as a diabetic. Even if you have taken to heart all the information piled on your lap thus far about diet and exercise, it means nothing if you see it all as a pointless drudge. The best medicine is your positive, forward-thinking attitude.

Here are three steps that will bring out the active and motivated person in you:

1. Start with an exercise plan—a diet, a regimen, an exercise routine, any of the things we have covered thus far. Try anything reasonable that your doctor recommends.
2. Follow that plan for at least the next six months.
3. After six months pass, work on your plan with new strategies that you learn as you go. What are the things you need to change? What parts of your personal campaign against the disease do you need to enhance? Keep changing, keep growing, and never, ever stop.

There might be factors at play here that aren't your fault. Only certain things in your life as a diabetic are within your control, as with any illness. Perhaps the timing was wrong. Maybe you didn't have enough information or advice to work with. Many diet and exercise regimens collapse within two to four weeks, often because people are missing the expert insight needed to ensure that these lifestyle changes stick. This is why it is important to establish your own personal health care team. A home-brewed, haphazard effort can at times be as counterproductive as no effort at all. Professional advice keeps you organized and motivated.

Fitness experts and nutritionists who guide you toward your exercise goals are only half the equation, as all the advice in the world won't help if you are unwilling to follow through. The dedication that turns good ideas into a healthier life can only come from you. Familial stress or pressure alone simply doesn't cut it, because then you are obviously changing yourself only to please others. You have to constantly ask what it is you want for yourself, not what someone else wants for you, the patient. As you begin to trust your choices over time, the distance between your challenges and your goals narrows, and former obstacles seem more like guideposts.

THE HEALTHY LIFESTYLE

The road to better health is paved with motivation, self–control, and a positive outlook. Don't worry about whether you can accomplish your goals or not. As long as you can keep a picture in your mind of where you want to go and how you are going to get there, you won't be disappointed in the results.

It is really as simple as this: to lose a pound, you have to burn 3,500 calories. To gain a pound, you have to eat 3,500 calories. In short, losing weight is all about doing more and consuming less. You never overfill your car's gas tank, so why overfill your stomach? That would be wasteful. Neither does it make sense to eat calories and let them go to waste—or to your *waist*.

It is very important to remember the factors that lead to diabetes, because if you forget, you won't be able to avoid them at all, even with all the motivation in the world. Below is an effective strategy for a healthy lifestyle as a diabetic:

- Learn about carbohydrates, proteins, fats, and balancing your meals.
- Engage in physical activity every day.
- Learn proper portion sizing.
- Use the plate method to balance meals and control portions.

- Keep a diary of what you eat.
- Maintain a neat and tidy dining and cooking environment.
- Learn the medical basis for hunger and how to control it.
- Eat and drink in moderation.
- Don't live your life around the bathroom scales.
- Plan your meals for the entire week.
- Eat more fruits and vegetables.
- If you are a smoker, then quit. If you aren't, then avoid taking up this damaging habit.

JOURNALING YOUR WAY THROUGH DIABETES

Never forget that you are your own greatest ally and supporter. If you can't trust yourself to back you up in times of need, diabetes or not, then who *can* you trust?

One way that you can add structure to your cause is through journaling. Keep a record of the things you do and experience, whom you talk to and why, what you feel about them, and so on. Journaling puts you under the microscope in a good way, since no one is pressuring you to be the next Earnest Hemingway. No one but you will ever see your writing, unless you want to reveal it to someone. Inscribe elegant prose in your finest calligraphy, or just scribble in pencil. All that matters is that you write what's on your mind and in your heart.

Alternatively, what if you want the whole world to see what you are thinking? Why not post an online journal in the form of a blog or share your experiences and insights on one of the many networking sites? What you are going through and how you are going through it matters above all. What you share might well be a lifeline to another diabetic who is going through a crisis. Of course, ongoing communication with friends and family, through phone, correspondence, and e-mail is essential both to your own health and the well-being of others.

You can also join online support groups, which allows you to meet people who are sharing their own issues and feelings about diabetes.

READING FOR YOUR OWN GOOD

Can you survive a day, or even an hour, without a book in your hand? If not, you may possess one of the strongest personal skills there is in the fight against diabetes. Your love of books is like having a secret weapon. Knowledge really is power.

Recipe books, diabetes journals, and books of any and all genres, from yoga practice to gardening, can provide vital information, support, and inspiration. You can research many of these books online or spend an hour or two browsing in your local library, where you may very well find just what you want. Having medical information at your fingertips is one of the most powerful components in the war on diabetes.

CONNECT WITH OTHER MOTIVATED PEOPLE

Staying motivated and energized on your own is difficult, but you can always use your own personal interests to help you. When you join a focus health group, you forge bonds, exchange ideas, and stay excited about your healthier lifestyle. Visit local groups in your area to see if one is right for you, or take advantage of an online group. There are like-minded people from all over the world waiting to meet you there. Simply put, a voyage is easier and more fulfilling if you have friends to share it with.

STICKING TO THE PLAN IN SPITE OF RESTRICTIONS

Diabetes can rob you of some of the basic pleasures in life, but there is still no need to think of your condition as some torture device. Every door closed is a window opened, and if you look carefully and keep an open mind, you will discover ways to enjoy yourself and be healthy too.

Imagine a special occasion, like a birthday party for a friend or loved one. What do you do? You can't celebrate things the way you used to if you have diabetes. Or can you? With some creativity and imagination, you can participate in any social event without violating your health restrictions.

Here are some useful ideas for special occasions:

1. If you are hosting a party, plan the courses or refreshments the same way you would if you were preparing for yourself. Remember that it is really not about a "diabetic meal plan," but rather it is about eating healthily from a generalized scope. For appetizers, you can serve bruschetta, stuffed grape leaves, lettuce wraps, sushi rolls, crackers, antipasto, artichoke hearts, pickled asparagus, or raw veggies with a light dip. There is an endless list of things you can serve without

overstepping your dietary boundaries or leaving your guests feeling as though they are being forced to accommodate your condition. For the main course, try vegetarian and ethnic dishes, as found in Indian and Asian cuisine. For dessert, why not serve a fruit salad with thin, crispy cookies or a pudding topped with raspberry sauce? Who says you can't live life and eat healthily at the same time?

2. If you are invited to a potluck or similar event, you can bring a nutritious, diabetic-friendly treat of your own to the occasion. You can explain to your friends and family that eating healthily can be a very exciting experience.

3. Holidays like Thanksgiving and Christmas are often marked by elaborate feasts, which can leave diabetics sadly out in the cold. It can be a demotivating experience to set turkey and stuffing off limits. Who says you can't prepare a feast on your own terms? Just like in the above examples, you can prepare a delicious and healthy dinner for your family and friends and still contribute to a joyful occasion. You can fight your cravings, avoid being left out, and stay motivated all at the same time.

4. Try not to miss any meals. This can throw your metabolism way off balance and will spoil a holistic plan. Once you deviate from a permanent schedule, it can be difficult to get it back.

5. Remember that it *is* possible to have too much of a good thing. Overindulging is an unhealthy habit, regardless of how healthy the food is. Follow these strategies to keep motivated, but don't forget to portion your meals when you eat.

MOTIVATION TO GO

Staying motivated is difficult because the simple act of living is saddled with rules on diet, activities, and other aspects of life that most people take for granted. Nowhere on that list, however, is there any kind of restriction against seeing the world. Even with diabetes, there is nothing stopping you from traveling the globe, but before you go, consider the following.

Pay your physician a visit. Have your vitals screened and your blood tested a few days ahead of your flight. Make sure your glucose levels are as much under control as possible. If you take insulin or other medications and you have plans for air travel or are leaving the country, obtain a letter from your doctor describing your condition and outlining the medical precautions you require. If you need vaccinations, take care of them several weeks before your departure, as sometimes vaccinations can have adverse effects on your diabetes control. You will also need to know how to adjust your glucose levels and take insulin medications yourself if you are traveling alone. Be sure of what supplies you need to take with you so that you are prepared to handle your diabetes wherever you are in the world.

The more you understand that you can travel with diabetes, the more unrestricted you will feel.

SLEEP: ANOTHER MOTIVATIONAL AGENT

In our modern world of never-ending work, "sleep is weak" is a common motto, and an unhealthy one at that. Sleep is a vital requirement, like eating and breathing, especially when your body needs to keep functioning at full efficiency throughout the day. Getting enough sleep is important for staying alert and energetic, so you can begin each day at your best. However, like all of the other topics we have covered, there are things to do, and not to do, regarding sleep.

Drinking a couple of espressos after watching the evening news is a recipe for a night of insomnia. Assuming you get to sleep at all, you will wake up tense and irritable the next morning. A better idea would be a warm bath with Epsom salts, which relax muscles and stimulate the production of serotonin and melatonin, chemical triggers that relieve anxiety and prepare the body for sleep.

Research indicates that the only hours of sleep that really count are the ones just before and shortly after midnight. You need to adjust your hours accordingly and take into account what kind of environment helps you fall asleep. Can you sleep with the lights on? Can you sleep with the lights off? Decide what is best for you and stick to it.

SEEKING INSPIRATION

Finding the right inspiration to fix your diabetes can be a wearisome thing to do on your own. Health groups and social communities can guide you toward being healthier, but you may be drawn to seek the answers to deeper questions about life.

The idea of God or a higher power transcends religion or cultural distinction. Regardless of what label you apply to yourself, if you know there is someone out there to whom you can turn in times of need, you have a reason to keep moving forward.

Life with diabetes is often a struggle and can feel like an uphill climb. As you pass through difficult stretches, you may be tempted to surrender, feeling that you have done everything you can. You may seek advice from your loved ones, perhaps even a professional therapist, and they all tell you to keep faith and stay positive.

Well, can you?

Are you willing to pin your hopes on a brighter tomorrow that you can't really see yet? No doctor would ever prescribe prayer, but it can help you to get things off your chest instead of letting them wear you down emotionally. If you feel you need God's help to carry on through trying times, tell him.

Faith can be a powerful force in life for some diabetics. Things happen all the time that reason alone cannot explain. You hear the common phrase "everyday miracles," but the point is that they can happen to anyone, including yourself. You have nothing to lose and much to gain. Many health book authors found their way to wellness through a transformative experience that they believe came from a higher power or deity.

You don't have to leave home to go on a spiritual journey. Just disconnect yourself from rational concerns for a short while and find a new perspective on life. Spirituality can provide both peace and a moral center. It is more than just an individual experience; it is a way to reach out to other diabetics.

Even if you consider yourself a reasonable being, or you simply do not feel like following a more spiritual path at present, inspiration can pour down on you from all directions. Inspiration can come in the form of a child's smile, a rainbow, and all the little wonders that hint at the presence of something greater than us.

FINDING MEANING THROUGH SELF-MOTIVATION,
SELF-PLANNING, AND MORE

What gives your life meaning? How happy are you with your life right now? Are you satisfied with what you have, or do you dwell on what you don't?

If you continue to think positively and dedicate yourself to changing your life and health for the better, you can improve yourself by finding meaning in everything you do and everything you experience.

How do you find balance in your life? Your spiritual side can provide this answer. Self-motivation is not a label or a brand name belonging to a particular religion. Self-motivation is universal and personal, accessible to one and all, and yet unique to every individual. It is the part that you plan out all by yourself. You use it to find the strength to face the challenges ahead.

Self-motivation is the core of what makes you who you are. How you see the world affects how you react to it. With diabetes, the world tends to look much smaller and bleaker. Things that once made sense don't seem so realistic anymore. Things you once took for granted are gone, and the life ahead of you may appear full of needless suffering.

You may find yourself asking questions like these:

- Why me?
- Why my family?
- Why this?
- Will this go on forever?
- Why do bad things happen to good people?
- How can I face my life?
- How can I face this illness?

Alcoholics Anonymous and drug rehab centers recognize the power of self-motivation to help people break their bad habits and gear themselves toward improvement.

However, this is not to say that you can use your future goals as a crutch to lean on. Your plans must be converted into action. To regard self-motivation as the sole and infallible avenue of your triumph over diabetes is foolish and destructive. Improving your life and your health must take both self-planning *and* effort on your part.

Self-motivation and self-planning can provide solace for patients who suffer from pain or chronic illness. Proper self-motivation teaches us that illness is not a punishment brought on by some moral failing, real or imagined, but a mere consequence of biology.

The mind and body are more connected than most people imagine, and there are many who claim that they were indeed healed through faith in defiance of scientific explanation. Wherever you find motivation, it is a way to improve yourself, perhaps through a direct channel to divine intervention. There is no arguing against the benefits of belief. Through your own self-motivation, you can make sense of your life and your health. If you can find meaning in your life, you can better handle the emotional and physical challenges ahead of you.

Ironically, as the world population continues to grow, families shrink, and people live their lives more distantly. Many grow despondent without the extensive support networks of friends and relatives that existed in the past. This change forces us to seek out our own means of encouragement. Often this means challenging previous assumptions about what is important in life. Things certainly look different after sorting them out and prioritizing.

Material gain is a driving force for many people, including diabetics. The pursuit of wealth, social grandeur, and status symbols, combined with the emotional upheaval that diabetes brings, may convince some patients to seek an expensive modern miracle that will stamp out their illness and let them return to their previous way of living. The lucky ones will take a different lesson from their past experiences and find something more essential to cherish. Remember that you are still in charge of your life, no matter what the situation.

Staying focused, finding faith, and taking charge of your life are all ways that you can find the motivation needed to achieve your goals.

Every once in a while, when the road stretches on out of sight, you may wonder what would happen if you took a little shortcut. You might cut corners on your diet, bending the rules a little, indulging in things you ordinarily are not entitled to, and thinking that a minor infraction might as well not be an infraction at all. The problem is that bad habits tend to be repetitive. That's why they are called habits, not actions. You think that if you got away with it once, you can get away with it again and again, and before long, your entire motivational plan falls apart.

Medical discipline and self-control are of supreme value here. You would be driving without a steering wheel without them. If you continue to ignore diabetic guidelines designed to lead you to better health, it will be impossible to get better. Moreover, you lose sight of why things are not improving the way they should.

In the end, you are the only one who can tell you what to do. If you decide it is too much effort, that you would rather be overweight than actually work at improving your health, you are well within your rights to do so. However, don't get bogged down by pessimism. You will be amazed at what you can accomplish with nothing more than a positive attitude; and spiritual guidance will help to give you the perspective you need to jump whatever hurdles life puts in your way.

Once you have established this can-do mind-set, the rest of the journey is an easy downhill ride. Keep it up, and conquering diabetes will be a snap.

Lastly, meditation is another gateway for many who prefer to find strength in themselves. Focus and pay attention to the present moment, and let your inner self make a few of the decisions for you. Let your mind and body be one, and shut out the distractions of the world around you. This is how to really unleash the strength and motivation needed to pursue a better and healthier life as a diabetic.

Glossary

acanthosis nigricans. A condition of the human body characterized by the appearance of dark, thickened, velvety patches in the armpit, groin, and back of neck. This may be due to insulin resistance.

amylopectin. A complex sugar characterized by a highly branched glucose chain, mostly found in plants.

angina pectoris. A crushing and severe pain in the chest region. The condition is characterized also by a feeling of suffocation and pressure just under the breastbone due to the absence of an adequate supply of oxygen to the muscles of the heart.

angiotensin. A family of peptides that are smaller than proteins. Their main function is to constrict the blood vessels, and they are known as vasoconstrictors.

appendectomy. Surgical removal of the appendix.

atherogenic. Pertaining to the initiation or increase of atherogenesis, which is the process of depositing lipids and calcium in the arterial lumen.

Avandia. A type of drug that is generally prescribed for the treatment of Type 2 diabetes.

C-reactive protein. A special type of plasma protein whose concentration is known to increase with the presence of any inflammation in the body.

catecholamines. An amine derived from the amino acid tyrosine. There are many disorders that involve the catecholamines, such as neuroblastoma, pheochromocytoma, and so on.

chronic disease. A disease that lasts three months or more. The term *chronic* comes from the Greek term *chronos*, which means "long lasting."

chylomicrons. Substances found in the lymphatic and cardiovascular system made up of proteins and lipids.

191

claudication. Pain or cramping in the lower portion of the leg as a result of inadequate blood supply to the muscles. The word is derived from the Latin word *claudicare*, meaning "to limp."

Coxsackie virus. A family of enteroviruses, first discovered in the town of Coxsackie near the southern region of Albany, New York. These viruses are divided into two types: A and B. The A type is associated with hand, foot, and mouth disease. These viruses are associated with juvenile diabetes.

Crohn's disease. A chronic inflammatory disease mainly affecting the intestines. The disease also affects the digestive system.

dialysis. A special process by which the body is purged of the waste products that accumulate when the kidneys are malfunctioning. The dialysis machine takes over the function of the human kidneys.

disaccharide. A carbohydrate formed by the combination of two monosaccharides, or simple sugars.

endocrinologist. A physician who specializes in the diagnosis and treatment of the diseases that affect the endocrine system.

exocrine. A type of gland that secretes its contents with the help of a duct.

glucagon. A hormone secreted by the pancreas. This hormone increases sugar levels, acting in reverse of the effect of insulin.

gluconeogenesis. The process of synthesizing glucose from noncarbohydrate sources.

glycemic index. A very important indicator of the ability of food materials that contain carbohydrates to increase blood sugar levels within a period of two hours. Food materials containing carbohydrates that break down very quickly have a high glycemic index.

glycogen. The most common form in which body glucose is stored.

glycogenesis. The process by which glycogen is formed from glucose.

glycolysis. A process involving the breakdown of glucose or other carbohydrates in the absence of oxygen to release energy. The by-product of this reaction in human beings is lactic acid.

Goodpasture's syndrome. A disease affecting the lungs and the kidneys. It is autoimmune in nature. Bleeding in the lungs is one of the main symptoms of this disease.

hemochromatosis. This term, meaning "iron overload," is a very common genetic disorder among Caucasians. In this disease, the body tends to retain more iron than it requires.

herniation. The abnormal protrusion of tissues through an opening in the body.

high-density lipoprotein. The form in which lipids are generally transported from one area of the body to another. High-density lipoproteins, or

HDL, transport cholesterol from the tissues to the liver in order to help in its excretion through bile.

hyperglycemia. The condition of high sugar (glucose) levels in the blood. Sustained hyperglycemia may lead to diabetes.

hyperkalemia. Elevated potassium levels. Potassium is one of the major elements of the body. The proper level of potassium is very essential for ordinary functioning.

hyperlipidemia. A condition in which there is an excess of fats or lipids in the bloodstream.

hyperosmolar coma. A condition of coma caused by an abnormal increase of osmolar concentration.

hyperosmolar hyperglycemic nonketotic syndrome (HHNS). A very complicated condition in which the blood glucose level becomes very high, resulting in severe dehydration of the body. If untreated, this may lead to diabetic coma.

intron. An essential part of a gene that is transcribed into the primary RNA transcript. These are also known as intervening sequences.

islets of Langerhans. Special cells present within the pancreas that are involved in the secretion of hormones, especially insulin.

lacto-ovo vegetarians. People who do not want to eat any kind of meat but are open to eating dairy and egg products.

low-density lipoprotein. The form in which cholesterol is transported from the liver to the various tissues of the body. The low-density lipoproteins, or LDLs, are generally referred to as "bad cholesterol."

Lyme disease. A disease caused by bacteria from the Spirochete genus. The disease may result in abnormalities in the skin, joints, heart, and nervous system.

macrovascular disease. Disease of the large blood vessels, including the coronary arteries and the aorta.

metformin. A common drug often referred to as the first line of defense against Type 2 diabetes.

microalbuminuria. A state of slight elevation in the excretion of protein albumin through the urine. The presence of this protein is not detected by the conventional assay.

microangiopathy. A condition in which the walls of small blood vessels become very thick and weak. The walls of the vessels start to leak blood and protein, and in the process the blood flow is also slowed down.

microvascular disease. Disease of the finer blood vessels of the body, including the capillaries.

monosaccharide. The most basic form of carbohydrate that is very important for the sustenance of any organism. It is the simplest form of sugar and is colorless, crystalline, and water soluble. Common examples are glucose, fructose, and galactose.

nephropathy.   Any damage to or disease of the kidney. Generally, the specific cause of the disease is placed just before this term.

neuropathic pain.   A very severe pain that may be the result of an injury sustained by the nervous system. The injury can be either to the central nervous system or to the peripheral nervous system.

pathophysiology.   The condition in which the normal functioning of an individual or an organ is hampered due to disease.

phytochemicals.   Chemicals that occur naturally in plants. The best example of a phytochemical is beta-carotene.

polydipsia.   The condition in which a person feels excessive thirst.

polyglandular autoimmune syndrome.   A genetic autoimmune disease that is associated with many clinical features, including underfunctioning of the parathyroid glands, yeast infection, and malfunctioning of the adrenal glands.

polyuria.   An excessive passage of urine. It can reach up to 2.5 liters per day for an adult.

preproinsulin.   A polypeptide molecule made of 110 amino acids. Preproinsulin becomes proinsulin, which in turn is converted to insulin.

renal.   Anything related to kidneys. For example, renal arteries are arteries in the kidney.

retinopathy.   Any kind of noninflammatory disease in the retina of the eye. The specific cause of the disease is placed just before this term, for instance *diabetic retinopathy*.

rosiglitazone.   A type of drug used to treat patients with Type 2 diabetes.

tachycardia.   A condition in which the heart beats faster than normal. Under this condition, the heart rate is more than one hundred beats per minute.

therapeutic.   The part of medicine concerned with the treatment of various diseases. For example, the therapeutic dosage of a medicine is the amount of that medicine required to treat a given disease or ailment.

thyroidectomy.   The surgical removal of part or all of the thyroid gland. This operation is done to remove a tumor from the gland or as part of the treatment for hyperthyroidism.

urticaria.   Another name for the common disease known as hives. This is characterized by raised, itchy areas of the skin and may well be a sign of an impending allergic reaction.

vagus nerve.   A mixed nerve in contact with most parts of the abdominal viscera, including the pharynx, larynx, lungs, heart, esophagus, and stomach.

Resources

Diabetes Research Institute
200 S. Park Road, Suite 100
Hollywood, FL 33021
(800) 321-3437
Fax: (954) 964-7036
info@drif.org

Juvenile Diabetes Research Foundation International (JDRF)
26 Broadway, 14th Floor
New York, NY
(800) 533-CURE (2873)
Fax: (212) 785-9595
info@jdrf.org
www.jdrf.org

University of Chicago DRTC
Donald Steiner, M.D., or Graeme Bell, Ph.D.
Howard Hughes Medical Institute
5841 S. Maryland Ave., AMB N216
Chicago, IL 60637
(773) 702-1334
Fax: (773) 702-4292
dfsteine@uchicago.edu

Vanderbilt University DRTC
Alvin C. Powers, M.D.
Joe C. Davis Chair in Biomedical Science
802 Light Hall
Nashville, TN 37232
(615) 322-7004
Fax: (615) 343-0172
al.powers@vanderbilt.edu

Albert Einstein College of Medicine DRTC
Elizabeth A. Walker, Ph.D.
1300 Morris Park Ave.
Belfer Building, Room 705
Bronx, NY 10461
(718) 430-3242
Fax: (718) 430-8557
walker@aecom.yu.edu

Washington University DRTC
Edwin Fisher, Ph.D.
4444 Forest Park Ave.
St. Louis, MO 63108
(314) 286-1900 or 1940
Fax: (314) 286-1919
efisher@im.wustl.edu

Indiana University DRTC
David G. Marrero, Ph.D.
250 N. University Blvd., Room 122
Indianapolis, IN 46202
(317) 278-0905
Fax: (317) 278-0911
dgmarrer@iupui.edu

Applied Diabetes Research Inc.
1420 Valwood Pkwy.
Carrollton, TX 75006
(972) 241-1884
www.applieddiabetesresearch.org

The Jackson Laboratory—Diabetes
600 Main St.

Bar Harbor, ME 04609
(207) 288-6000
www.jax.org/diabetes

Scripps Whittier Diabetes Institute
9894 Genesee Ave.
La Jolla, CA 92037
(877) WHITTIER (944-8843)
Fax: (858) 626-5680
www.scripps.org/services/diabetes

DIABETES ENDOCRINOLOGY RESEARCH CENTERS (DERCS)

Yale University School of Medicine DERC
Robert Sherwin, M.D.
P.O. Box 208020
333 Cedar St.
New Haven, CT 06520-8020
(203) 785-4183
Fax: (203) 737-5558
robert.sherwin@yale.edu
www.info.med.yale.edu/intmed/faculty/sherwin.html

University of Washington DERC
Jerry P. Palmer, M.D.
DVA Puget Sound Health Care System
1660 S. Columbian Way
Seattle, WA 98108
(206) 764-2688
Fax: (206) 764-2693
jpp@u.washington.edu
www.depts.washington.edu/diabetes

University of Pennsylvania DERC
Mitchell Lazar, M.D.
415 Curie Blvd.
Philadelphia, PA 19104
(215) 898-0198
Fax: (215) 898-5408
lazar@mail.med.upenn.edu
www.uphs.upenn.edu/endocrin/faculty/lazar.html

University of Massachusetts Medical School DERC
Aldo Rossini, M.D.
373 Plantation St., Suite 218
Worcester, MA 01605
(508) 856-3800
Fax: (508) 856-4093
Aldo.Rossini@umassmed.edu
www.umassmed.edu/diabetes

University of Iowa DERC
Robert Bar, M.D.
3E19 VA Medical Center
Iowa City, IA 52246
(319) 338-0581, ext. 7625
Fax: (319) 339-7025
robert-bar@uiowa.edu
www.int-med.uiowa.edu/faculty.html

University of Colorado DERC
John Hutton, Ph.D.
1775 N. Ursula St.
P.O. Box 6511, Mail Stop Box B-140
Aurora, CO 80045
(303) 724-6837
Fax: (303) 724-6838
john.hutton@uchsc.edu
www.uchsc.edu/misc/diabetes/DERC

Massachusetts General Hospital DERC
Joseph Avruch, M.D.
55 Fruit St.
Boston, MA 02114
(617) 726-6909
Fax: (617) 726-6909
avruch@molbio.mgh.harvard.edu

Joslin Diabetes Center DERC
C. Ronald Kahn, M.D.
1 Joslin Place
Boston, MA 02215
(617) 732-2635

Fax: (617) 732-2487
c.ronald.kahn@joslin.harvard.edu
www.joslin.harvard.edu

DIABETES ORGANIZATIONS

World Health Organization (WHO)
Daniel Epstein
(202) 974-3459
epsteind@paho.org
www.who.int/diabetes

U.S. Department of Health and Human Services—U.S. Food and Drug Administration (FDA)
10903 New Hampshire Ave.
Silver Spring, MD 20993
(888) INFO-FDA (463-6332)

National Institute of Diabetes and Digestive and Kidney Diseases (NIDDK)
National Diabetes Information Clearinghouse (NDIC)
1 Information Way
Bethesda, MD 20892
(800) 860-8747
Fax: (703) 738-4929
ndic@info.niddk.nih.gov
www.diabetes.niddk.nih.gov

Central Ohio Diabetes Association
1100 Dennison Ave.
Columbus, OH
(614) 884-4400 or 4484
coda@diabetesohio.org

American Diabetes Association (ADA)
1701 N. Beauregard St.
Alexandria, VA 22311
Call center: (800) DIABETES (342-2383)
Service center: (703) 549-1500

Fax: (703) 549-6995
askada@diabetes.org
membership@diabetes.org
www.diabetes.org

Diabetes Exercise and Sports Association (DESA)
310 W. Liberty, Suite 604
Louisville, KY 40202
(800) 898-4322
Fax: (502) 581-0206
www.diabetes-exercise.org

American Diabetes Association for Information Memorials
1701 N. Beauregard St., Suite 100
Alexandria, VA 22311
(800) 342-2383
askada@diabetes.org

The Hormones Foundation
8401 Connecticut Ave., Suite 900
Chevy Chase, MD 20815
(800) HORMONE (467-6663)
Fax: (301) 941-0259
hormone@endo-society.org
www.hormone.org/diabetes

American Heart Association—The "Heart of Diabetes" Program
7272 Greenville Ave.
Dallas, TX 75231
review.personal.info@heart.org
(800) AHA-USA1 (242-8721)

Diabetes Exercise and Sports Association (DESA)
8001 Montcastle Dr.
Nashville, TN 37221
(800) 898-4322
Fax: (615) 673-2077
desa@diabetes-exercise.org
www.diabetes-exercise.org

International Diabetes Federation
Chaussée de la Hulpe 166
B-1170 Brussels, Belgium
+32-2-5385511★
+32-2-5385114
info@idf.org
www.idf.org

Diabetics in the Area of Waycross Gathering for Support (D.A.W.G.S.)
Diabetes Support Group
Waycross, GA
(912) 283-6086
Fax: (413) 674-6480
croberts77@gmail.com
www.livingwellwithdiabetes.org

National Glycohemoglobin Standardization Program (NGSP)
Randie R. Little, Ph.D.
1 Hospital Dr., N712
Columbia, MO 65212
(573) 882-6882
Fax: (573) 884-8823
ngsp@missouri.edu
www.ngsp.org

Friends with Diabetes International
31 Herrick Ave., Unit B
Spring Valley, NY 10977
(845) 352-7532
Fax: (845) 573-9276
webmaster@friendswithdiabetes.org
www.friendswithdiabetes.org

Diabetes Research and Wellness Foundation
5151 Wisconsin Ave., NW, Suite 420
Washington, DC
(202) 298-9211
Fax: (202) 244-4999
diabeteswellness@diabeteswellness.net
www.diabeteswellness.net

Diabetes Action Research and Education Foundation
426 C St., NE
Washington, DC
(202) 333-4520
Fax: (202) 558-5240
info@diabetesaction.org
www.diabetesaction.org

NATIONALLY RECOGNIZED DIABETES CLINICS

Huguley Memorial Medical Center
11801 South Freeway
Fort Worth, TX
(817) 551-2706
www.huguley.org

Indian Health Service National Diabetes Program
5300 Homestead Rd., NE
Albuquerque, NM 87110
(505) 248-4182 or 4236
Fax: (505) 248-4188
diabetesprogram@mail.ihs.gov
www.ihs.gov/medicalprograms/diabetes

Veterans Health Administration (VHA)
Program Chief, Diabetes
810 Vermont Ave., NW
Washington, DC 20420
(202) 273-5400
Fax: (202) 273-9142
www.va.gov/diabetes/#veterans

Bayer Diabetes Care Center
555 White Plains Rd.
Tarrytown, NY 10591

The Mayo Clinic—Diabetes
Ginger Plumbo
(507) 284-5005

plumbo.ginger@mayo.edu
www.mayoclinic.org/diabetes

Rice Diabetes Center
4004 82nd St.
Lubbock, TX
(806) 722-3110
Fax: (806) 722-3115

Diabetes Centers of America
7863 Callaghan Rd., #206
San Antonio, TX
(210) 525-1206

Centers for Diabetes Management
24048 Highway 59 North
Kingwood, TX
(281) 358-3387

DRI Kosow Diabetes Treatment Center
(305) 243-6504
Clinical research: (305) 243-6145
Course registration: (305) 243-1062
info@drif.org
www.drif.org

Abbott Diabetes Care Inc.
1360 South Loop Rd.
Alameda, CA 94502

Diabetes America
15200 Southwest Freeway, #360
Sugar Land, TX
(832) 237-3500

Juvenile Diabetes Research Foundation
6836 San Pedro Ave.
San Antonio, TX 78216
(210) 829-1919
Fax: (210) 822-1443

Centegra Diabetes Center
360 Station Dr.
Crystal Lake, IL 60014
(815) 356-2382
www.centegra.org/cpc

Sequoia Hospital Diabetes Institute
170 Alameda De Las Pulga,
Redwood City, CA 94062
(650) 367-5213
www.sequoiahospital.org/Medical_Services/Diabetes_Center

University of California School of Medicine, Diabetes Center
500 Parnassus Ave.
San Francisco, CA 94122
(415) 353-2266

Sanford Diabetes Care Center
1305 W. 18th St.
Sioux Falls, SD 57104
(800) 445-5788
info@sanfordhealth.org
www.sanfordhealth.org

McLeod Regional Medical Center—Diabetes Center
555 E. Cheves St.
Florences, SC 29506
(843) 777-2000

Self-Management Diabetes Center
617 W. Pierce St.
Carlsbad, NM 88220
(575) 887-8141

California Diabetes Program
California Department of Public Health
1616 Capitol Ave., Suite 74.420
Sacramento, CA 95814
(916) 552-9888
Fax: (916) 552-9988
www.caldiabetes.org

Winchester Medical Center Diabetes Management
2 Medical Plaza Dr., 105
Winchester, VA 22601
(540) 536-5108
www.valleyhealthlink.com

Berkshire Medical Center—Diabetes Program
725 North St.
Pittsfield, MA 01201
(413) 395-7942

Children's Diabetes Foundation at Denver
777 Grant St., Suite 302
Denver, CO 80203
(303) 863-1200
www.childrensdiabetesfdn.org

Mercy Diabetes Center
910 N. Eisenhower Ave.
Mason City, IA 50401
(800) 443-3883

Cotton-O'Neil Diabetes and Endocrinology Center
3520 SW 6th Ave.
Topeka, KS 66606
(785) 354-9591
www.stormontvail.org

Skaggs Diabetes and Endocrinology Care
545 Branson Landing Blvd.
Branson, MO 65616
(417) 348-8990
www.skaggs.net

Helene Fuld Medical Center—Diabetes Treatment Center
750 Brunswick Ave.
Trenton, NJ 08618
(609) 394-6694

Seminole Nation—Indian Diabetes Program
12574 Ns. 3540

Seminole, OK 74868
(405) 382-3761

Raleigh Community Hospital—Diabetes Treatment Center
3400 Wake Forest Rd.
Raleigh, NC 27609
(919) 876-3185

Forsyth Medical Center Diabetes and Nutrition Services
1900 S. Hawthorne Rd., Suite 504
Winston-Salem, NC 27103
(336) 277-1660
www.forsythmedicalcenter.org

St. Margaret Diabetes and Endocrine Center
815 Freeport Rd.
Pittsburgh, PA 15215
(412) 784-4950
www.stmargaret.upmc.com

Utah Valley Diabetes Management Clinic
1134 N. 500 West, #103
Provo, UT 84604
(801) 357-7546

Intermountain Cottonwood Endocrine and Diabetes Center
5770 S. 250 East, #310
Salt Lake City, UT 84107
(801) 314-4500
Fax: (801) 314-2909

Sky Lakes Diabetes Service
2865 Daggett Ave.
Klamath Falls, OR
(541) 274-2633
www.skylakes.org

Albany Memorial Hospital—Diabetes Treatment Center
600 Northern Blvd.
Albany, NY 12204
(518) 471-3500

New York Diabetes Center
2649 Strang Blvd.
Yorktown Heights, NY 10598
(914) 248-4000

Diabetes and Lipid Clinic of Alaska
2841 Debarr Rd., #43
Anchorage, AK 99508
(907) 274-7847
www.diabetesalaska.com

Northwest Diabetes Life Skills Center
7492 N. La Cholla Blvd.
Tucson, AZ 85741
(520) 742-2121

Humphreys Diabetes Center
1226 W. River St.
Boise, ID 83702
(208) 331-1155
www.hdiabetescenter.org

Diabetes Awareness and Service Center
614 E. Emma Ave.
Springdale, AR 72764
(479) 756-8758

International Diabetes Center
3800 Park Nicollet Blvd.
St. Louis Park, MN 55416
(888) 825-6315
Fax: (952) 993-1302
www.parknicollet.com

DIABETES EDUCATION AND TRAINING

American Association of Diabetes Educators (AADE)
200 W. Madison Ave., Suite 800
Chicago, IL 60606
(800) 338-3633

Fax: (312) 424–2427
aade@aadenet.org
www.diabeteseducator.org

TCOYD (Taking Control of Your Diabetes)
1110 Camino Del Mar, Suite B
Del Mar, CA 92014
(800) 99–TCOYD (998-2693)
Fax: (858) 755-6854
info@tcoyd.org
www.tcoyd.org

National Diabetes Education Program (NDEP)
1 Diabetes Way
Bethesda, MD 20814
(800) 438-5383
Fax: (703) 738-4929
ndep@mail.nih.gov
www.ndep.nih.gov

Centers for Disease Control and Prevention (CDC)
Division of Diabetes Translation
Mail Stop K-10
4770 Buford Highway, NE
Atlanta, GA 30341-3717
(800) CDC-INFO (232-4636)
Fax: (770) 488-8211
diabetes@cdc.gov
www.cdc.gov/diabetes

Diabetes Action Research and Education Foundation
426 C St., NE
Washington, DC 20002
(202) 333-4520
Fax: (202) 558-5240
info@diabetesaction.org
www.diabetesaction.org

Diabetes Resource Center Inc.
1944 Braselton Hwy., 104/207

Buford, GA 30519
(800) 354-0004
www.diabetesresourcecenter.org

Diabetes Education Center
7100 Oakmont Blvd.
Fort Worth, TX 76132
(817) 370-5990

Diabetes Self Management Education
6200 W. Parker Rd.
Plano, TX 75093
(972) 981-8116

Diabetes Health Consulting Inc.
16810 W. U.S. Hwy. 82
Muenster, TX 76252
(940) 768-8120

Blake Medical Center—Diabetes Education Program
2020 59th St. West
Bradenton, FL 34209
(941) 798-6134
www.blakemedicalcenter.com

JFK Medical Center—Diabetes Education Center
5301 S. Congress Ave.
Atlantis, FL 33462
(561) 733-7286

University Community Hospital—Diabetes Education
3100 E. Fletcher Ave.
Tampa, FL 33602
(813) 615-7620
www.uch.org

Augusta Medical Center—Diabetes Education
78 Medical Center Dr.
Staunton, VA 24401
(540) 213-2537
www.augustamed.com

Diabetes Education and Care
15 W. 65th St.
New York, NY 10023
(212) 712-9944
www.jgb.org

Dupont Hospital Diabetes Education Program
2520 E. Dupont Rd.
Fort Wayne, IN 46825
(260) 416-3260

Hendricks Diabetes Self Management Skills Training Center
3937 Ferrara Drive
Silver Spring, MD 20906
(301) 942-0678

Mount Nittany Medical Center—Diabetes Education
1800 E. Park Ave.
State College, PA 16803
(814) 231-7095

Diabetes Educators
170 N. 1100 East
American Fork, UT 84003
(801) 763-3463

Diabetes Education Center of Arizona
3522 N. 3rd Ave.
Phoenix, AZ 85013
(480) 941-7363

Diabetes Education and Camping Association (DECA)
P.O. Box 385
Huntsville, AL 35804
(256) 230-0619
Fax: (256) 230-3171
www.diabetescamps.org

Council for the Advancement of Diabetes Research and Education (CADRE)
320 7th Ave., Box 291

Brooklyn, NY 11215
(718) 766-8799
Fax: (718) 360-1324
cadre@cadre-diabetes.org
www.cadre-diabetes.org

Crawford Diabetes Educational
701 10th St., SE
Cedar Rapids, IA 52403
(319) 398-6711

DIET-RELATED DIABETES RESOURCES

Ifood.tv—Diabetes
Media contact: media@ifood.tv
Content partnership: content@ifood.tv
General inquiries: admin@ifood.tv
www.ifood.tv/network/diabetic_candy_bar/recipes

Recipe Zaar
www.recipezaar.com/recipes/diabetic

Natural Diabetes Control
info@naturaldiabetics.com
www.naturaldiabetics.com/tag/sugar-replacement

Diabetic Diet Meals
http://diabetesinfocenter.org (search term: Diabetes Diet)

Desserts for Diabetics
eHow Inc.
15801 NE 24th St.
Bellevue, WA 98008
www.ehow.com (search term: Diabetic Desserts)

Diabetic Gourmet Magazine
CAPCO Marketing
8417 Oswego Rd., #177
Baldwinsville, NY 13027
www.diabeticgourmet.com

DIABETES Q AND A

Familydoctor.org
http://familydoctor.org (search term: Diabetes)
AnswersTV
400 W. Erie St.
Chicago, Il 60654
(312) 421-0113
contactus@answerstv.com

Yahoo Answers: Diabetes
http://answers.yahoo.com (search term: Diabetes)

AOL Health: Diabetes
www.thediabetesblog.com

DIABETES PRODUCTS AND SUPPLIES

Life Clinic (Diabetes Personal Health Management Products)
Lifeclinic International Inc.
4032 Blackburn Lane
Burtonsville, MD 20866
(301) 476-9888
Fax: (301) 476-9388

Medicool Inc. Diabetes Health and Beauty
20460 Gramercy Place
Torrance, California 90501
(800) 433-2469
Fax: (310) 427-7274
www.medicool.com

Lifeclinic International Inc.
7855 Division Dr.
Mentor, OH 44060
(800) 543-2787
Fax: (931) 967-4891
service@lifeclinic.com
www.lifeclinic.com

Abbott Diabetes Care Products
1360 South Loop Rd.
Alameda, California 94502
abbottdiabetescare.com
(888) 522-5226
FreeStyle Navigator (glucose monitor) 24-hour product support: (866) 597-5520

Advanced Diabetics Solutions
1314 Texas St.
Houston, TX 77002
(713) 222-2270
www.advanceddiabeticsolutions.net

Diabetic Shoes Hub LLC
13256 N. 93rd Way
Scottsdale, AZ 85260
(623) 455-6258
support@diabeticshoeshub.com

Healthy Feet Store
7965 Dunbrook Rd., Suite C
San Diego, CA 92126
(858) 547-8800
Fax: (858) 547-8812
www.healthyfeetstore.com/diabeticshoes.html

Goods Diabetic Supplies
14601 Marsha Dr.
Mesquite, TX 75180
(972) 557-0972

MedCare Inc. Diabetic Supplies
902 Clint Moore Rd., Suite 214
Boca Raton, FL 33487
(800) 407-0109
Fax: (877) 866-2664
www.discountdiabeticsupplies.com

Western Diabetic Supply
1140 36th St.

Ogden, UT 84403
(801) 622-4339
www.westerndiabetic.com

The Candy Gift Basket
5723 Pierson Mountain Ave.
Longmont, CO 80503
(866) 732-8130
customersupport@thecandygiftbasket.com
www.thecandygiftbasket.com/product/a-diabetic

Diabetic Candy.com Inc.
P.O. Box 775
Yaphank, NY 11980
(888) 420-2277
judy@diabeticcandy.com
www.diabeticcandy.com

Ayurgold Blood Sugar Regulation
17th Ave. South, #3
Nampa, ID 83651
English: (800) 721-6301
Other languages: (800) 721-0650

DexCom Inc.
6340 Sequence Dr.
San Diego, CA 92121
(858) 200-0200
Fax: (858) 200-0201
info@dexcom.com
www.dexcom.com

Diabeat Natural Herbs
+86 21 50599398, ext. 805
Fax: +86 21 50599398, ext. 801
bianyitcmx@hotmail.com
www.diabeat.cc

Diabetes Solutions
422 Austin Ave.
Geneva, IL 60134
(630) 262-1573

FREE MATERIALS FOR DIABETICS

Free Diabetes Identification Necklaces
Diabetes Research and Wellness Foundation
5151 Wisconsin Ave., NW, Suite 420
Washington, DC 20016
(202) 298-9211
Fax: (202) 244-4999
diabeteswellness@diabeteswellness.net
www.diabeteswellness.net
(Click on the necklace link at the bottom of the page.)

Diabetic Symptoms Alert:
www.free-symptoms-of-diabetes-alert.com

Xubex: Free Diabetes Kits and Supplies
MCS Enterprises Inc.
P.O. Box 1244
Winter Park, FL 32790
(866) 699-8239
Fax: (407) 671-7960
www.xubex.com/FDK.aspx

Free Glucometers
www.diabeticsupplyinc.com

Free Diabetes Testing Supplies—Medicare
Liberty Medical Supply
10400 South Federal Hwy.
Port St. Lucie, FL 34952
(866) 331-6559

Free Diabetes Cookbooks
www.totallyfreestuff.com/index.asp?ID=26683
www.lifeclinic.com/whatsnew/cookbook/DiabetesCookbook.asp

The Cochrane Library (free virtual diabetes library)
www.cochrane.org (search term: Diabetes)

The Diabetes Digest (free diabetes magazine)
diabetesdigest.com/DD_subscription.htm

ADDITIONAL DIABETES RESOURCES AND WEBSITES

WebMD
2300 Wilson Blvd., #600
Arlington, VA 22201
(703) 302-1040
Fax: (703) 248-0830
comments@thcn.com
www.diabetes.webmd.com

List of Diabetes Care Specialists
Health Grades Inc.
500 Golden Ridge Rd., Suite 100
Golden, CO 80401

Health Line—Diabetes
www.healthline.com/hlbook/action-plan-for-diabetes

Diabetes Daily
www.diabetesdaily.com

Diabetes in Control
Dave Joffe—Editor in Chief
editor@diabetesincontrol.com
www.diabetesincontrol.com

How Stuff Works: Diabetes
1 Capital City Plaza
3350 Peachtree Rd., Suite 1500
Atlanta, GA 30326
(404) 760-4729
www.health.howstuffworks.com/diabetes.htm

Health Central—Diabetes
www.healthcentral.com/diabetes/find-drug.html

NIH Diabetes Senior Health
custserv@nlm.nih.gov
http://nihseniorhealth.gov/diabetes/toc.html

Endocrine Web—Diabetes
www.endocrineweb.com/diabetes

Diabetic Books
www.diabeticsbooks.com

Diabetes Monitor
info@diabetesmonitor.com
www.diabetesmonitor.com

Insulin Manufacture
www.madehow.com/Volume-7/Insulin.html

Childhood Diabetes Resources
www.childdiabetes.org
www.kidsource.com/kidsource/content/insulin.html
www.childrenwithdiabetes.com

Diabetes Success Stories
www.aolhealth.com/condition-center/diabetes/success-stories
www.naturaldiabetics.com/diabetes-success-stories
www.forecast.diabetes.org/magazine/features/diabetes-success-stories

Diabetes Forecast (magazine from the American Diabetes Association)
Attention: Editor
1701 N. Beauregard St.
Alexandria, VA 22311
forecasteditor@diabetes.org

References

CHAPTER 1

Alexander, G., N. Sehgal, R. Moloney, and R. Stafford. 2008. National trends in treatment of type 2 diabetes mellitus, 1994–2007. *Archives of Internal Medicine* 168 (19): 2088–94.

American Diabetes Association. 2008. *All about diabetes.* diabetes.org/about-diabetes.jsp.

Anderson, J. E. 2006. A patient with type 2 diabetes and cirrhosis of the liver. *Clinical Diabetes* (24): 43–44.

Anonymous. 1965. Diabetes: A scope monograph on the nature, diagnosis, and treatment of diabetes mellitus. Kalamazoo, MI: Upjohn Company.

Bennett, J. C., and F. Plum, eds. 1996. *Cecil textbook of medicine.* 20th ed. Philadelphia: W. B. Saunders.

Busse, F. P., P. Hiermanna, A. Gallera, M. Stumvollb, T. Wiessnerb, W. Kiessa, and T. Kapellena. 2007. Evaluation of patients' opinion and metabolic control after transfer of young adults with type 1 diabetes from a pediatric diabetes clinic to adult care. *Hormone Research* 67 (3): 132–38.

Centers for Disease Control and Prevention, CDC. 2005. National diabetes fact sheet: General information and national estimates on diabetes in the United States. Atlanta, GA: U.S. Department of Health and Human Services.

Ceriello, A., and S. Colagiuri. 2008. International Diabetes Federation guideline for management of postmeal glucose: A review of recommendations. *Diabetic Medicine* 25 (10): 1151–56.

Crea, R., A. Kraszewski, T. Hirose, and K. Itakura. 1978. Chemical synthesis of genes for human insulin. *Proceedings of the National Academy of Sciences* 75 (12): 5765–69.

Dean, L. 2004. *Introduction to diabetes.* National Center for Biotechnology Information website. ncbi.nlm.nih.gov/bookshelf/br.fcgi?book=diabetes&part=A5.

Fowler, M. J. 2008. Hypoglycemia. *Clinical Diabetes* 26:170–73.

Frank, R. N. 2004. Diabetic retinopathy. *New England Journal of Medicine* 350 (1): 48–58.

Harris, E. H. 2005. Elevated liver function tests in type 2 diabetes. *Clinical Diabetes* 23:115–19.

Hilsted, J. 1982. Pathophysiology in diabetic autonomic neuropathy: Cardiovascular, hormonal, and metabolic studies. *Diabetes* 31:730–37.

Imura, H. 2000. Diabetes: Current perspectives. *New England Journal of Medicine* 342:1533.

Isselbacher, K., E. Braunwald, J. Wilson, J. Martin, A. Fauci, and D. Kasper, eds. 1994. *Harrison's principles of internal medicine.* 13th ed. New York: McGraw-Hill.

Lefebvre, P. 2002. Diabetes yesterday, today and tomorrow: Work of the International Federation of Diabetes. *Bulletin et Memoires de l'Academie Royale de Medecine de Belgique* 157 (10–12): 455–63.

Macleod, J. 1925. *Insulin: Its use in the treatment of diabetes.* Baltimore, MD: Williams and Wilkins.

Marks, J. B. 2003. Clinical diabetes and the diabetes epidemic. *Clinical Diabetes* 21:2–3.

MoveForward. 2009. The alarming statistics on diabetes. Diabetes Forum website. diabetesforum.com/blog/2009/06/the-alarming-statistics-on-diabetes.

National Geographic Society. 1998. *National Geographic eyewitness to the 20th century.* Washington, DC: National Geographic Society.

Peters, A. 2005. *Conquering diabetes: A complete program for prevention and treatment.* New York: Plume.

Reaven, G. M. 1988. Banting lecture: Role of insulin resistance in human disease. *Diabetes* 37:1595–1607.

Serri, O. 1991. Somatostatin analogue, octreotide, reduces increased glomerular filtration rate and kidney size in insulin-dependent diabetes. *Journal of the American Medical Association* 265 (7): 888–92.

Shro, R. J. 2004. Case study: Screening and treatment of prediabetes in primary care. *Clinical Diabetes* 22:98–100.

Smeltzer, S., and B. Bare. 2004. *Medical-surgical nursing.* Vol. 1. 10th ed. (Philippine). Philadelphia: Lippincott.

Smeltzer, S., and B. Bare. 2004. *Medical-surgical nursing.* Vol. 2. 10th ed. (Philippine). Philadelphia: Lippincott.

Stretton, A. 2002. The first sequence: Fred Sanger and insulin. *Genetics* 162 (2): 527–32.

Ward, W., J. Beard, J. Halter, M. Pfeifer, and D. Porte Jr. 1984. Pathophysiology of insulin secretion in non–insulin-dependent diabetes mellitus. *Diabetes Care* 7:491–502.

Williamson, R. T. 1898. *Diabetes mellitus and its treatment.* London: Pentland.

Wilson, M. 2008. *Carbohydrates, proteins, and fats.* Merck website. merck.com/mmhe/sec12/ch152/ch152b.html.

CHAPTER 2

American Diabetes Association. 2004. Hyperglycemic crises in diabetes. Clinical practice recommendations. *Diabetes Care* 27 (Suppl. 1): S94–S102.

American Diabetes Association. 2007. Type 2 Diabetes. Author website. www.diabetes
.org/type-2-diabetes.jsp.

Aronovitz, M., and B. Metzger. 2006. Gestational diabetes mellitus. In D. C. Dale and
D. D. Federman, eds., *ACP Medicine*, sec. 9, chap. 4. New York: WebMD.

Bell, D., and J. Alele. 1997. Diabetic ketoacidosis: Why early detection and aggressive
treatment are crucial. *Postgraduate Medical Journal* 101 (9): 193–200.

Buchanan, T., A. Xiang, S. Kjos, and R. Watanabe. 2007. What is gestational diabetes? *Diabetes Care* 30 (Suppl. 2): S105–S111.

Buse, J., K. Polonsky, and C. Burant. 2008. Type 2 diabetes mellitus. In P. R. Larsen
et al., eds., *Williams Textbook of Endocrinology*, 11th ed., 1329–81. Philadelphia:
Saunders Elsevier.

Capell, P. 2004. Case study: Hemachromatosis in type 2 diabetes. *Clinical Diabetes*
22:101–102.

Diabetes in Control. 2005. *New type 3 diabetes discovered.* Author website. diabetesin
control.com/index.php?option=com_content&view-article&id=2582.

De Felice, F., M. Vieira, T. Bomfim, H. Decker, P. Velasco, M. Lambert, K. Viola,
W.-Q. Zhao, S. Ferreira, and W. Klein. 2009. Protection of synapses against
Alzheimer's-linked toxins: Insulin signaling prevents the pathogenic binding of Aβ
oligomers. *Proceedings of the National Academy of Sciences* 106 (18): 7678.

Peters, A. 2005. *Conquering diabetes: A complete program for prevention and treatment.* New
York: Plume.

Robertson, G. L. 2003. What is diabetes insipidus? Diabetes Insipidus Foundation Inc.
website. www.diabetesinsipidus.org/whatisdi.htm.

Smeltzer, S., and B. Bare. 2004. *Medical-surgical nursing.* Vol. 2. 10th ed. (Philippine).
Philadelphia: Lippincott.

Steenhuysen, J. 2009. Insulin protects brain from Alzheimer's: U.S. study. UK Reuters
website. http://uk.reuters.com/article/idUKN0253100820090202.

CHAPTER 3

Allen C., T. LeCaire, M. Palta, K. Daniels, M. Meredith, and D. D'Alessio. 2001.
Risk factors for frequent and severe hypoglycemia in type 1 diabetes. *Diabetes Care*
24 (11): 1878–81.

American Diabetes Association. 2004. Smoking and diabetes: Clinical practice recommendations 2004. *Diabetes Care* 27 (Suppl. 1): S74–S75.

American Diabetes Association. 2008. The genetics of diabetes. Author website. www
.diabetes.org/genetics.jsp.

Bristow, I. R., and M. C. Spruce. 2009. Fungal foot infection, cellulitis and diabetes:
A review. *Diabetic Medicine* 26 (5): 548–51.

Clarke W., L. Gonder-Frederick, F. Richards, and P. Cryer. 1991. Multifactorial origin of hypoglycemic symptom unawareness in IDDM: Association with defective
glucose counterregulation and better glycemic control. *Diabetes* 40:680–85.

Cryer, P. E. 2004. Diverse causes of hypoglycemia-associated autonomic failure in diabetes. *New England Journal of Medicine* 350 (22): 2272–79.

Ganda, P. 1980. Pathogenesis of macrovascular disease in the human diabetic. *Diabetes* 29:931–42.

Giovannucci, E., E. Rimm, M. Stampfer, G. Colditz, and W. Willett. 1998. Diabetes mellitus and risk of prostate cancer (United States). *Cancer Causes and Control* 9 (1): 3–9.

Harjutsalo, V., S. Katoh, C. Sarti, N. Tajima, and J. Tuomilehto. 2004. Population-based assessment of familial clustering of diabetic nephropathy in Type 1 diabetes. *Diabetes* 53:2449–54.

Hawkins, M., and L. Rossetti. 2005. Insulin resistance and its role in the pathogenesis of type 2 diabetes. In *Joslin's Diabetes Mellitus*, 14th ed., 425–48. Philadelphia: Lippincott.

Jones, M., R. Drut, M. Valencia, and A. Mijalovsky. 2005. Empty sella syndrome, panhypopituitarism, and diabetes insipidus. *Fetal and Pediatric Pathology* 24 (3): 191–204.

Liu, S., S. Chen, K. Chang, and J. Wang. 2004. Brain abscess presenting as postpartum diabetes insipidus. *Taiwanese Journal of Obstetrics and Gynecology* 43 (1): 46–49.

Mayo Clinic staff. October 11, 2008. Diabetes symptoms: When to consult your doctor. Mayo Clinic website. mayoclinic.com/health/diabetes-symptoms/DA00125.

Medical News Today. 2006. Type 1 diabetes: Worldwide study looks to find causes. www.medicalnewstoday.com/articles/37702.php.

Remuzzi, G., A Schieppati, and P. Ruggenenti. 2002. Clinical practice: Nephropathy in patients with type 2 diabetes. *New England Journal of Medicine* 346 (15): 1145–51.

Schoenstadt, A. 2008. Symptoms of diabetes. EMedTV website. http://diabetes .emedtv.com/diabetes/symptoms-of-diabetes.html.

Smeltzer, S., and B. Bare. 2004. *Medical-surgical nursing.* Vol. 2. 10th ed. (Philippine). Philadelphia: Lippincott.

Smyth, D., V. Plagnol, N. Walker, J. Cooper, K. Downes, J. Yang, J. Howson, H. Stevens, R. McManus, C. Wijmenga, G. Heap, P. Dubois, D. Clayont, J. Hunt, D. van Heel, and J. Todd. 2008. Shared and distinct genetic variants in type 1 diabetes and celiac disease. Pub Med website. www.ncbi.nlm.nih.gov/pubmed/19073967.

Tabibiazar, R., and S. Edelman. 2003. Silent ischemia in people with diabetes: A condition that must be heard. *Clinical Diabetes* 21 (1): 5–9.

Takasawa, H., Y. Takahashi, M. Abe, K. Osame, S. Watanabe, T. Hisatake, K. Yasuda, Y. Kaburagi, H. Kajio, and M. Noda. 2007. An elderly case of type 2 diabetes which developed in association with oral and esophageal candidiasis. *Internal Medicine* 46 (7): 387–89.

Tintinalli, J., D. Gabor, and J. Stapczynski. 2003. *Emergency medicine: A comprehensive study guide.* 6th ed. New York: McGraw-Hill Professional.

Willis, J. 2009. *Causes of diabetes.* Sclero website. www.sclero.org/medical/symptoms/ associated/diabetes/causes.html.

Zochodne, D. W. 2001. Peripheral nerve disease. In H. C. Gerstein, R. B. Haynes, eds., *Evidence-based diabetes care*, 466–87. Hamilton, ON: B. C. Decker.

CHAPTER 4

American Diabetes Association. 2001. Postprandial blood glucose. *Clinical Diabetes* 19:127–30.

American Diabetes Association. 2004. Retinopathy in diabetes: Clinical practice recommendations 2004. *Diabetes Care* 27 (Suppl. 1): S84–S87.

American Diabetes Association. 2008. Standards of medical care in diabetes—2008. *Diabetes Care* 31:S12–S54.

Clement, S., S. Braithwaite, M. Magee, A. Ahmann, E. Smith, R. Schafer, and I Hirsch. 2004. Management of diabetes and hyperglycemia in hospitals. *Diabetes Care* 27:553.

Cox, M., and D. Edelman. 2009. Tests for screening and diagnosis of type 2 diabetes. *Clinical Diabetes* 27:132–38.

Masharani, U., and M. German. 2007. Pancreatic hormones and diabetes mellitus. In D. G. Gardner et al., eds., *Greenspan's basic and clinical endocrinology*, 8th ed., 716–46. New York: McGraw-Hill.

Mitka, M. 2007. Poor patient adherence may undermine aim of continuous glucose monitoring. *Journal of the American Medical Association* 298 (6): 614–15.

National Diabetes Information Clearinghouse. 2008. Diagnosis of diabetes. Author website. http://diabetes.niddk.nih.gov/dm/pubs/diagnosis/index.htm.

Peters, A. 2005. *Conquering diabetes: A complete program for prevention and treatment.* New York: Plume.

Porcellati, F. 2003. Counterregulatory hormone and symptom responses to insulin-induced hypoglycemia in the postprandial state in humans. *Diabetes* 52 (11): 2774–83.

Sapountzi, P., G. Charnogursky, M. Emanuele, D. Murphy, F. Nabhan, and N. Emanuele. 2005. Case study: Diagnosis of insulinoma using continuous glucose monitoring system in a patient with diabetes. *Clinical Diabetes* 23:140–43.

Schrot, R., K. Patel, and P. Foulis. 2007. Evaluation of inaccuracies in the measurement of glycemia in the laboratory, by glucose meters, and through measurement of hemoglobin A1c. *Clinical Diabetes* 25:43–49.

Shlipak, M. 2008. Diabetic nephropathy. Online version of *BMJ Clinical Evidence.* www.clinicalevidence.com.

Smeltzer, S., and B. Bare. 2004. *Medical-surgical nursing.* Vol. 2. 10th ed. (Philippine). Philadelphia: Lippincott.

U.S. Preventive Services Task Force. 2008. *Screening for gestational diabetes mellitus.* www.ahrq.gov/clinic/uspstf/uspsgdm.htm.

CHAPTER 5

American Diabetes Association. 2004. Clinical practice recommendations 2002. *Diabetes Care* 27:51.

American Diabetes Association. 2006. Pancreas and islet transplantation in type 1 diabetes: Position statement. *Diabetes Care* 29 (4): 935.

American Diabetes Association. 2008. Standards of medical care in diabetes. Clinical practice recommendations 2008. *Diabetes Care* 31 (Suppl. 1): S3–S110.

Briscoe, V., and S. Davis. 2006. Hypoglycemia in type 1 and type 2 diabetes: Physiology, pathophysiology, and management. *Clinical Diabetes* 24:115–21.

Cheng, A. Y. Y., and B. Zinman. 2005. Principles of insulin therapy. In *Joslin's Diabetes Mellitus*, 14th ed., 659–70. Philadelphia: Lippincott.

Decker, S., C. Burt, and J. Sisk. 2009. Trends in diabetes treatment patterns among primary care providers. *Journal of Ambulatory Care Management* 32 (4): 333–41.

Fowler, M. J. 2009. Inpatient diabetes management. *Clinical Diabetes* 27:119–22.

Gabbe, S., and C. Graves. 2003. Management of diabetes mellitus complicating pregnancy. *Obstetrics and Gynecology* 102 (4): 857–68.

Guthrie, R. 2001. Is there a need for a better basal insulin? *Clinical Diabetes* 19:66–70.

Hod, M., and Y. Yogev. 2007. Goals of metabolic management of gestational diabetes. *Diabetes Care* 30 (Suppl. 2): S180–S187.

Peters, A. 2005. *Conquering diabetes: A complete program for prevention and treatment.* New York: Plume.

Pickup, J., and H. Keen. 2002. Continuous subcutaneous insulin infusion at 25 years. *Diabetes Care* 25 (30): 593–98.

Smeltzer, S., and B. Bare. 2004. *Medical-surgical nursing.* Vol. 2. 10th ed. (Philippine). Philadelphia: Lippincott.

Stevens, R., S. Matsumoto, and C. Marsh. 2001. Is islet transplantation a realistic therapy for the treatment of type 1 diabetes in the near future? *Clinical Diabetes* 19:51–60.

UK Prospective Diabetes Study Group. 1998. Intensive blood-glucose control with sulphonylureas or insulin compared with conventional treatment and risk of complications in patients with type 2 diabetes UKPDS 33. *Lancet* 352:461–62.

Van Acker, K., D. De Bacquer, S. Weiss, K. Matthys, H. Raemen, C. Mathieu, and I. Colin. 2009. Prevalence and impact on quality of life of peripheral neuropathy with or without neuropathic pain in type 1 and type 2 diabetic patients attending hospital outpatients clinics. *Diabetes and Metabolism* 35 (3): 206–13.

Vernon, M., and J. Eberstein. 2004. *Atkins diabetes revolution.* New York: HarperCollins.

White, J., and R. Campbell. 2001. Recent developments in the pharmacological reduction of blood glucose in patients with Type 2 diabetes. *Clinical Diabetes* 19:153–59.

White, J., S. Davis, R. Cooppan, M. Davidson, K. Mulcahy, G. Manko, D. Nelinson, and the Diabetes Consortium Medical Advisory Board. 2003. Clarifying the role of insulin in type 2 diabetes management. *Clinical Diabetes* 21:14–21.

White, S., R. James, S. Swift, R. Kimber, and M. Nicholson. 2001. Human islet cell transplantation: Future prospects. *Diabetic Medicine* 18 (2): 78–103.

CHAPTER 6

American Diabetes Association. 2004. Diabetes care in the school and day care setting: Clinical practice recommendations 2004. *Diabetes Care* 27 (Suppl. 1): S122–S128.

Arterberry, M., K. Cain, and S. Chopko. 2007. Collaborative problem solving in five-year-old children: Evidence of social facilitation and social loafing. *Educational Psychology* 27 (5): 577–96.

Cain, K., C. Dweck, and G. Heyman. 1992. Young children's vulnerability to self-blame and helplessness. *Child Development* 63 (2): 401–15.

Copeland, K., D. Becker, M. Gottschalk, and D. Hale. 2005. Type 2 diabetes in children and adolescents: Risk factors, diagnosis, and treatment. *Clinical Diabetes* 23:181–85.

Dweck, C. 2006. *Mindset*. New York: Random House.

Dweck, C., and P. Smiley. 1994. Individual differences in achievement goals among young children. *Child Development* 65 (6): 1723–43.

Erdley, C., K. Cain, C. Loomis, F. Dumas-Hines, and C. Dweck. 2007. Relations among children's social goals, implicit personality theories, and responses to social failure. *Developmental Psychology* 33 (2): 263–72.

Harris, M., D. Mertlich, and J. Rothweiler. 2001. Parenting children with diabetes. *Diabetes Spectrum* 14 (4): 182–84.

Hviid, A., M. Stellfeld, J. Wohlfahrt, and M. Melbye. 2004. Childhood vaccination and type 1 diabetes. *New England Journal of Medicine* 350 (14): 1398–1404.

Juvenile Diabetes Research Foundation International. 2007. Monogenic diabetes. Author website. monogenicdiabetes.org/whatis.html.

Kamins, M., and C. Dweck. 1999. Person vs. process praise and criticism: Implications for contingent self-worth and coping. *Developmental Psychology* 35:835–47.

Kirpichnikov, D., S. McFarlane, and J. Sowers. 2002. Metformin: An update. *Annals of Internal Medicine* 137:25.

Levetan, C. 2001. Into the mouths of babes: The diabetes epidemic in children. *Clinical Diabetes* 19:102–4.

Levine, B., B. Anderson, D. Butler, J. Antisdel, J. Brackett, and L. Laffel. 2001. Predictors of glycemic control and short term adverse outcomes in youth with type 1 diabetes. *Journal of Pediatrics* 139 (2): 197–203.

Northam, E., D. Rankins, A. Lin, R. Wellard, G. Pell, S. Finch, G. Werther, and F. Cameron. 2009. Central nervous system function in youth with Type 1 diabetes 12 years after disease onset. *Diabetes Care* 32:445–50.

Rapaport, W. 1998. *When diabetes hits home: The whole family's guide to emotional health*. Alexandria, VA: American Diabetes Association.

Renukuntla, V., K. Hassan, S. Wheat, and R. Heptulla. 2009. Disaster preparedness in pediatric type 1 diabetes mellitus. *Pediatrics* 124 (5): e973–77.

Rewers, A., P. Chase, T. Mackenzie, P. Walravens, M. Roback, M. Rewers, R. Hamman, and G. Klingensmith. 2002. Predictors of acute complications in children with type 1 diabetes. *Journal of the American Medical Association* 287 (19): 2511–18.

Rosenbloom, A., and J. Silverstein. 2003. *Type 2 diabetes in children and adolescents*. Alexandria, VA: American Diabetes Association.

Rothman, R., S. Mulvaney, T. Elasy, T. Gebretsadik, A. Shintani, A. Potter, W. Russell, and D. Schlundt. 2008. Self-management behaviors, racial disparities, and glycemic control among adolescents with type 2 diabetes. *Pediatrics* 121 (4): e912–19.

Silverstein, J., G. Klingensmith, K. Copeland, L. Plotnick, F. Kaufman, L. Laffel, L. Deeb, M. Grey, B. Anderson, L. Holzmeister, and N. Clark. 2005. Care of children and adolescents with type 1 diabetes. *Diabetes Care* 28 (1): 186–212.

Travis L., B. Brouhard, and B. Schreiner. 1987. *Diabetes mellitus in children and adolescents.* Philadelphia: W. B. Saunders.

Vernon, M., and J. Eberstein. 2004. *Atkins diabetes revolution.* New York: HarperCollins.

CHAPTER 7

Davis, B., and T. Barnard. 2003. *Defeating Diabetes: A No-Nonsense Approach to Type 2 Diabetes and the Diabesity Epidemic.* United States: Healthy Living Publications.

Defeat Diabetes Foundation. 2009. Dementia meds increase risk for hyperglycemia in older diabetics. www.defeatdiabetes.org/news/view.asp?catid=&subcatid=&id=56675.

Defeat Diabetes Foundation. 2007. Depression Increases Diabetes Risk. Author website. www.defeatdiabetes.org/news/view.asp?catid=&subcatid=&id=36955.

Defeat Diabetes Foundation. 2008. Mental health linked to amputation risk in diabetes. Author website. www.defeatdiabetes.org/news/view.asp?catid=4009&subcatid=&id=43109.

DeNoon, D. 2009. *Diabetes slows brain function.* WebMD website. http://diabetes.webmd.com/news/20090105/diabetes-slows-brain-function.

Fisher, L., M. Skaff, J. Mullan, P. Arean, R. Glasgow, and U. Masharani. 2008. A longitudinal study of affective and anxiety disorders, depressive affect and diabetes distress in adults with Type 2 diabetes. *Diabetic Medicine* 25 (9): 1096–1101.

Funnell, M. M. 2006. The diabetes attitudes, wishes, and needs (DAWN) study. *Clinical Diabetes* 24:154–55.

Goldberg, R. W., B. Cooke, and A. Hackman. 2007. Mental health providers' involvement in diabetes management. *Psychiatric Services* 58:1501–2.

Gonzalez, J. S., S. Safren, L. Delahanty, E. Cagliero, D. Wexler, J. Meigs, and R. Grant. 2008. Symptoms of depression prospectively predict poorer self-care in patients with type 2 diabetes. *Diabetic Medicine* 25 (9): 1102–7.

Gregg, E. W., and A. Brown. 2003. Cognitive and physical disabilities and aging-related complications of diabetes. *Clinical Diabetes* 21:113–18.

Leichter, S. B., E. Dreelin, and S. Moore. 2004. Integration of clinical psychology in the comprehensive diabetes care team. *Clinical Diabetes* 22:129–31.

Lin, E., and M. Korff. 2008. Mental disorders among persons with diabetes: Results from the World Mental Health Surveys. *Journal of Psychosomatic Research* 65 (6): 571–80.

Llorente, M. D., and V. Urrutia. 2006. Diabetes, psychiatric disorders, and the metabolic effects of antipsychotic medications. *Clinical Diabetes* 24:18–24.

Osborn, D. P. 2008. Psychiatric disorders and diabetes mellitus. *British Journal of Psychiatry* 192:398.

Peters, A. 2005. *Conquering diabetes: A complete program for prevention and treatment.* New York: Plume.

Rapaport, W. 1998. *When diabetes hits home.* Alexandria, VA: American Diabetes Association.

Williams, M. M. 2006. Treating depression to prevent diabetes and its complications: Understanding depression as a medical risk factor. *Clinical Diabetes* 24:79–86.

Yeung, S., A. Fischer, and R. Dixon. 2009. Exploring effects of type 2 diabetes on cognitive functioning in older adults. *Neuropsychology* 23:1–9.

CHAPTER 8

American Diabetes Association. 2004. Hypertension management in adults with diabetes: Clinical practice recommendations 2004. *Diabetes Care* 27 (Suppl. 1): S65–S67.

American Diabetes Association. 2004. Influenza and pneumococcal immunization in diabetes: Clinical practice recommendations 2004. *Diabetes Care* 27 (Suppl. 1): S111–S113.

American Diabetes Association. 2004. Peripheral arterial disease in people with diabetes. *Clinical Diabetes* 22 (4): 181–89.

Bax, J., and E. Van der Wall. 2006. Assessment of coronary artery disease in patients with asymptomatic diabetes. *European Heart Journal* 27 (6): 631–32.

Boden, W., and D. Taggart. 2009. Diabetes with coronary disease: A moving target amid evolving therapies? *New England Journal of Medicine* 360:2570.

Davis, B., and T. Barnard. 2003. *Defeating diabetes: A no-nonsense approach to type 2 diabetes and the diabesity epidemic.* Summertown, TN: Healthy Living Publications.

Frye, R., P. August, M. Brooks, R. Hardison, S. Kelsey, J. MacGregor, T. Orchard, B. Chaitman, S. Genuth, S. Goldberg, M. Hlatky, T. Jones, M. Molitch, R. Nesto, E. Sako, and B. Sobel. 2009. For the BARI 2D study group: A randomized trial of therapies for type 2 diabetes and coronary artery disease. *New England Journal of Medicine* 360 (24): 2503.

Gerstein, H., K. Malmberg, S. Capes, and S. Yusuf. 2001. Cardiovascular disease. In H. C. Gerstein and R. B. Haynes, eds., *Evidence-based diabetes care*, 488–514. Hamilton, ON: B. C. Decker.

Grundy, S., J. Cleeman, S. Daniels, K. Donato, R. Eckel, B. Franklin, D. Gordon, R. Kraus, P. Savage, S. Smith Jr., J. Spertus, and F. Costa. 2005. Diagnosis and management of the metabolic syndrome: An American Heart Association/National Heart, Lung, and Blood Institute scientific statement. *Circulation* 112 (17): 2735–52.

Henry, R. R. 2001. Preventing cardiovascular complications of type 2 diabetes: Focus on lipid management. *Clinical Diabetes* 19:113–20.

Huxley, R., F. Barzi, and M. Woodward. 2006. Excess risk of fatal coronary heart disease associated with diabetes in men and women: Meta-analysis of 37 prospective cohort studies. *British Medical Journal* 332:73–78.

Lee, W., A. Cheung, D. Cape, and B. Zinman. 2000. Impact of diabetes on coronary artery disease in women and men: A meta-analysis of prospective studies. *Diabetes Care* 23 (7): 962–68.

Ludwig, D. S. 2002. The glycemic index: Physiological mechanisms relating to obesity, diabetes, and cardiovascular disease. *Journal of the American Medical Association* 287 (18): 2414–23.

Perkins, B., L. Aiello, and A. Krolewski. 2009. Diabetes complications and the renin-angiotensin system. *New England Journal of Medicine* 361 (1): 83–85.

Peters, A. 2005. *Conquering diabetes: A complete program for prevention and treatment.* New York: Plume.

Smeltzer, S., and B. Bare. 2004. *Medical-surgical nursing.* Vol. 2. 10th ed. (Philippine). Philadelphia: Lippincott.

Vernon, M., and J. Eberstein. 2004. *Atkins diabetes revolution.* New York: HarperCollins.

Wackers, F. 2005. Diabetes and coronary artery disease: The role of stress myocardial perfusion imaging. *Cleveland Clinic Journal of Medicine* 72 (1): 21–25.

Wood, R., J. Volek, S. Davis, C. Dell'Ova, and M. Fernandez. 2006. Effects of a carbohydrate-restricted diet on emerging plasma markers for cardiovascular disease. *Nutrition and Metabolism* 3:19.

Writing Team for the Diabetes Control and Complications Trial/Epidemiology of Diabetes Interventions and Complications Research Group. 2002. Effect of intensive therapy on the microvascular complications of type 1 diabetes mellitus. *Journal of the American Medical Association* 287:2563.

Zoler, M. L. 2008. CVD linked to diabetes, impaired glucose tolerance in older adults. *Family Practice News* 34 (24): 8.

CHAPTER 9

American Diabetes Association. 2000. Role of fat replacers in diabetes medical nutrition therapy: Clinical practice recommendations 2000. *Diabetes Care* 23 (Suppl. 1): S96–S97.

American Diabetes Association. 2003. Low-glycemic index diets in the management of diabetes: A meta-analysis of randomized controlled trials. *Diabetes Care* 26 (8): 2261–67.

American Diabetes Association. 2008. Nutrition recommendations and interventions for diabetes. *Diabetes Care* 31 (Suppl. 1): S61–S78.

Bogardus, C., E. Ravussin, D. Robbins, R. Wolfe, E. Horton, and E. Sims. 1984. Effects of physical training and diet therapy on carbohydrate metabolism in patients with glucose intolerance and non-insulin-dependent diabetes mellitus. *Diabetes* 33:311–18.

Byzzano, L., M. Serdula, and S. Liu. 2005. Prevention of type 2 diabetes by diet and lifestyle modification. *Journal of the American College of Nutrition* 24 (5): 310–19.

Campbell, A., and R. Beaser. 2007. Medical nutrition therapy. In R. S. Beaser et al., eds., *Joslin's Diabetes Deskbook*, 81–125. Boston: Joslin Diabetes Center.

Chalmers, K. H. 2005. Medical nutrition therapy. In C. R. Kahn et al., eds., *Joslin's Diabetes Mellitus*, 14th ed., 611–31. Philadelphia: Lippincott.

Davis, B., and T. Barnard. 2003. *Defeating diabetes: A no-nonsense approach to type 2 diabetes and the diabesity epidemic.* Summertown, TN: Healthy Living Publications.

Duarte-Gardea, M. 2004. Case study: The prevention of diabetes through diet and intense exercise. *Clinical Diabetes* 22:45–46.

Fung, T., M. McCullough, R. van Dam, and F. Hu. 2007. A prospective study of overall diet quality and risk of type 2 diabetes in women. *Diabetes Care* 30:1753–57.

Hippisley-Cox, J., and M. Pringle. 2004. Prevalence, care, and outcomes for patients with diet-controlled diabetes in general practice: Cross sectional survey. *Lancet* 364:423–28.

Hu, F., J. Manson, M. Stampfer, G. Colditz, S. Liu, C. Solomon, and W. Willett. 2001. Diet, lifestyle, and the risk of type 2 diabetes mellitus in women. *New England Journal of Medicine* 345 (11): 790–97.

Marks, J. B. 2004. The weighty issue of low-carbohydrate diets, or is the carbohydrate the enemy? *Clinical Diabetes* 22:155–56.

Parmet, S., C. Lynm, and R. Glass. 2006. Weight and diabetes. *Journal of the American Medical Association* 295 (11): 1330.

Peters, A. 2005. *Conquering diabetes: A complete program for prevention and treatment.* New York: Plume.

Saltmarch, N. R. 2001. Short diet plus modest lifestyle changes improve glucose tolerance. *Obesity, Fitness & Wellness Week*, September 8.

Vernon, M., and J. Eberstein. 2004. *Atkins diabetes revolution.* New York: HarperCollins.

CHAPTER 10

American Society of Pain Educators. 2006. Diabetic peripheral neuropathic pain: Consensus guidelines for treatment. *Journal of Family Practice* (Suppl. June): 3–19.

Britland, S., R. Young, A. Sharma, and B. Clarke. 1990. Association of painful and painless diabetic polyneuropathy with different patterns of nerve fiber degeneration and regeneration. *Diabetes* 39:898–908.

Daousi, C., I. McFalane, A. Woodward, T. Nurmikko, P. Bundred, and S. Benbow. 2004. Chronic painful peripheral neuropathy in an urban community: A controlled comparison of people with and without diabetes. *Diabetic Medicine* 21:976–82.

Davis, B., and T. Barnard. 2003. *Defeating diabetes: A no-nonsense approach to type 2 diabetes and the diabesity epidemic.* Summertown, TN: Healthy Living Publications.

Fishman, S., and L. Berger. 2000. *The war on pain.* New York: HarperCollins.

Galer, B., A. Gianas, and M. Jensen. 2000. Painful diabetic polyneuropathy: Epidemiology, pain description, and quality of life. *Diabetes Research and Clinical Practice* 47:123–28.

Hu, H. 1995. A review of treatment of diabetes by acupuncture during the past forty years. *Journal of Traditional Chinese Medicine* 15 (2): 145–54.

Kim, R., S. Edelman, and D. Kim. 2001. Musculoskeletal complications of diabetes mellitus. *Clinical Diabetes* 19:132–35.

Ko, G., N. Nowacki, L. Arseneau, M. Eitel, and A. Hum. 2010. Omega-3 fatty acids for neuropathic pain: Case series. *Clinical Journal of Pain* 26 (2): 168–72.

Lee, P., and R. Chen. 2008. Vitamin D as an analgesic for patients with type 2 diabetes and neuropathic pain. *Archives of Internal Medicine* 168 (7): 771–72.

National Diabetes Information Clearinghouse. Diabetic neuropathies: The nerve damage of diabetes. Author website. http://diabetes.niddk.nih.gov/dm/pubs/neuropathies/#body.

Obrosova, I. G. 2009. Diabetic painful and insensate neuropathy: Pathogenesis and potential treatments. *Neurotherapeutics* 6 (4): 638–47.

Otto, M., S. Bak, F. Bach, T. Jensen, and S. Sindrup. 2003. Pain phenomena and possible mechanism in patients with painful polyneuropathy. *Pain* 101:187–92.

Qiao, Q., S. Keinanen-Kiukaanniemi, U. Rajala, A. Uusimaki, and S. Kivela. 1995. Rheumatic pains of previously undiagnosed diabetic subjects. *Scandinavian Journal of Rheumatology* 24 (4): 234–37.

Raz, I., D. Hasdai, Z. Seltzer, and R. Melmed. 1988. Effect of hyperglycemia on pain perception and on efficacy of morphine analgesia in rats. *Diabetes* 37:1253–59.

Reichard, P., A. Britz, P. Carlsson, I. Cars, L. Lindblad, B. Nilsson, and U. Rosenqvist. 1990. Metabolic control and complications over 3 years in patients with insulin dependent diabetes IDDM: The Stockholm diabetes intervention study SDIS. *Journal of Internal Medicine* 228:511–17.

Rijken, P., J. Dekker, G. Lankhorst, K. Bakker, J. Dooren, and J. Rauwerda. 1998. Clinical and functional correlates of foot pain in diabetic patients. *Disability and Rehabilitation* 20 (9): 330–36.

Somers, D., and M. Somers. 1999. Treatment of neuropathic pain in a patient with diabetic neuropathy using transcutaneous electrical nerve stimulation applied to the skin of the lumbar region. *Physical Therapy* 79 (8): 767–75.

Sorensen, L., L. Molyneaux, and D. Yue. 2002. Insensate versus painful diabetic neuropathy: The effects of height, gender, ethnicity and glycemic control. *Diabetes Research and Clinical Practice* 57:45–51.

Vernon, M., and J. Eberstein. 2004. *Atkins diabetes revolution.* New York: HarperCollins.

Wong, M., J. Chung, and T. Wong. 2007. Effects of treatments for symptoms of painful diabetic neuropathy: Systematic review. *British Medical Journal* 335 (7610): 87.

Yoon, S., Y. Koga, I. Matsumoto, and E. Ikezono. 1987. An objective method of pulse diagnosis. *American Journal of Chinese Medicine* 14 (3–4): 179–83.

CHAPTER 11

Armstrong, N. 1987. Coping with diabetes mellitus: A full-time job. *Nursing Clinics of North America* 22 (3): 559–68.

Beck, M., B. Evans, H. Quarry-Horn, and J. Kerrigan. 2002. Type 2 Diabetes Mellitus: Issues for the medical care of pediatric and adult patients. *Southern Medical Journal* 95 (9): 992–1000.

Camach, F. 2002. Investigating correlates of health related quality of life in a low-income sample of patients with diabetes. *Quality of Life Research* 11 (8): 783–96.

Colberg, S. R. 2008. Encouraging patients to be physically active: What busy practitioners need to know. *Clinical Diabetes* 26:123–27.

Davis, B., and T. Barnard. 2003. *Defeating diabetes: A no-nonsense approach to type 2 diabetes and the diabesity epidemic.* Summertown, TN: Healthy Living Publications.

Delamater, A. M. 2006. Improving patient adherence. *Clinical Diabetes* 24:71–77.

Dovey-Pearce, G., R. Hurrell, C. May, C. Walker, and Y. Doherty. 2005. Young adults' 16–25 years suggestions for providing developmentally appropriate diabetes services: A qualitative study. *Health and Social Care in the Community* 13 (5): 409–19.

Fletcher, C. 1980. One way of coping with diabetes. *British Medical Journal* 280 (6222): 1115–16.

Funnell, M., and R. Anderson. 2004. Empowerment and self-management of diabetes. *Clinical Diabetes* 22:123–27.

Heisler, M., and K. Resnicow. 2008. Helping patients make and sustain healthy changes: A brief introduction to motivational interviewing in clinical diabetes care. *Clinical Diabetes* 26 (4): 161–65.

Huang, E., S. Gleason, R. Gaudette, E. Cagliero, P. Murphy-Sheehy, D. Natham, D. Singer, and J. Meigs. 2004. Health care resource utilization associated with a diabetes center and a general medicine clinic. *Journal of General Internal Medicine* 19 (1): 28–23.

Levensky, E. R. 2007. Motivational interviewing: An evidence-based approach to counseling helps patients follow treatment recommendations. *American Journal of Nursing* 107 (10): 50–58, quiz 58–59.

Lindahl, B. 2008. An illness behavior view on coping with diabetes. *International Journal of Behavioral Medicine* 15 (3): 165–66.

Madhu, K., and G. Sridhar. 2001. Coping with diabetes: A paradigm for coping with chronic illness. *International Journal of Diabetes in Developing Countries* 21 (2): 103–11.

Peters, A. 2005. *Conquering diabetes: A complete program for prevention and treatment.* New York: Plume.

Rapaport, W. 1998. *When diabetes hits home: The whole family's guide to emotional health.* Alexandria, VA: American Diabetes Association.

Tuchman, A. 2009. Diabetes and the public's health. *Lancet* 374:1140–41.

Index

maximum heart rate (MHR), 140
medications, heart attack risk lowering, 135
meditation, 122, 171
Mediterranean diet, 144, 211
meglitinide, 87, 89–90
metabolic syndrome, 15–16, 127, 129–31, 135–36, 138
metclopropamide, 92
metformin (Glucophage), 88, 96
metformin, 90, 92, 193
methionine, 134, 158
microalbumina, 26, 72, 193
microangiopathy, 50, 193
microvascular: disease, 193; complications, 49–50, 72
miglitol (Glyser), 89
mitochondria, 139
moderate hypoglycemia, 46
monogenic diabetes, 98
monoglycerides, 12
monosaccharides, 11, 193
monotherapy, 89
monounsaturated polyunsaturated fats, 222
Mount Sinai Medical Center, 33
multiple sclerosis, 38, 55
myocardial infarction, 49

nalidixic acid, 121
nateglinide, 90
NCEP (National Cholesterol Education Program), 131, 132, 191, 193, 195
nephrogenic DI, 34
neurodegeneration, 31
neurogenic Diabetes Insipidus, 34
neuropathy, 21, 23, 26, 42, 46, 49–50, 52–54, 75, 77, 80–81, 90–91, 164–66, 220, 224, 229–30; sensorimotor, 80; sudomotor, 54
neutral protamine Hagedorn (NPH), 82, 85
niacin, 135, 138
Niaspan, 135

NIDDM (Non-Insulin Dependent Diabetes Mellitus), 3, 220, 228
non-diet sodas, 156
nonstarchy vegetables, 228
Nordisk, 83
norepinephrine, 46
Norpramin, 167
nortriptyline (Pamelor), 166
Novolin: L, 82; N, 82–83; R, 82
nutrient depleted foods, 149
nutrient rich whole foods, 149
nutrient-starving heart symptoms, 49–50

O shape, 68
obesity, 23, 68, 129, 147
occlusive peripheral arterial diseases (PADs), 50
OGTT (Oral Glucose Tolerance Test), 57, 60–61
olive oil, 145
omega-3 fatty acids, 138–39, 169; long chain, 146
omega-6 fatty acids, 139
oral: alpha glucosidase inhibitors, 89; antidiabetic agents, 23, 59, 80, 90; antidiabetic medications, 87
orthostatic hypotension, 47, 63, 53
osmotic diuresis, 47, 48
osteoarthritis, 167
ovulation, 89
oxidative capacity, 17

pancreas: cells, 5, 9; cell transplants, 87; dysfunction, 13; functioning of, 13; islet cells, 87
panic attacks, 173
Panthenine, 138
pantothenic acid, 138
pathophysiological effects, 120
pathophysiology, 8, 40, 194, 220, 224
PCO_2 range, 71
PCOS (Polycystic Ovarian Syndrome), 64, 66–67

About the Author

Naheed Ali, M.D., has lectured at the Pennsylvania Institute of Technology. He has published more than 200 medically related articles for Suite 101 Media, Inc., an online magazine with more than 27 million visitors a month. Ali's articles (on politics, culture, and health) have been regularly featured on the home page of Worldpress.org, a topical news website boasting more than 300,000 readers monthly, and he has appeared as a health expert for *Weight Watchers* magazine, MSN Health, AOL News, and others. He is the author of *Are You Fit to Live?*

LaVergne, TN USA
15 March 2011
220118LV00002B/2/P